Essential Pharmacokinetics

A Primer for Pharmaceutical Scientists

For her love and support, this textbook is dedicated
to my wife, Hanna Lilja

Essential Pharmacokinetics

A Primer for Pharmaceutical Scientists

Thorsteinn Loftsson, PhD
Faculty of Pharmaceutical Sciences
University of Iceland
Reykjavik, Iceland

AMSTERDAM • BOSTON • HEIDELBERG • LONDON
NEW YORK • OXFORD • PARIS • SAN DIEGO
SAN FRANCISCO • SINGAPORE • SYDNEY • TOKYO

Academic Press is an imprint of Elsevier

Academic Press is an imprint of Elsevier
125 London Wall, London EC2Y 5AS, UK
525 B Street, Suite 1800, San Diego, CA 92101-4495, USA
225 Wyman Street, Waltham, MA 02451, USA
The Boulevard, Langford Lane, Kidlington, Oxford OX5 1GB, UK

Library of Congress Cataloging-in-Publication Data
A catalog record for this book is available from the Library of Congress.

British Library Cataloguing-in-Publication Data
A catalogue record for this book is available from the British Library.

ISBN: 978-0-12-801411-0

For Information on all Academic Press publications
visit our website at http://store.elsevier.com/

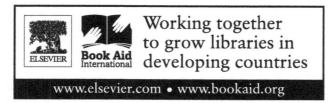

Working together
to grow libraries in
developing countries

www.elsevier.com • www.bookaid.org

Publisher: Mica Haley
Acquistion Editor: Kristine Jones
Editorial Project Manager: Molly McLaughlin
Production Project Manager: Caroline Johnson
Designer: Greg Harris

Typeset by MPS Limited, Chennai, India
www.adi-mps.com

Printed and bound in the United States of America

Contents

Preface

Pharmacokinetics is the study of drug kinetics within the body, including drug absorption, distribution, metabolism, and excretion. Pharmacokinetics is most commonly used in clinical situations to enhance the therapeutic efficacy of a patient's drug therapy. However, pharmacokinetics can also be applied in drug design and in the testing of formulations and novel drug delivery systems, as well as in quality evaluations of drug products. This book describes the mathematics used in the mammillary model, which is the most common compartmental model used in pharmacokinetics, and explains how pharmacokinetics can be applied in pharmaceutical product development. This book not only explains the basic concepts of pharmacokinetics and its clinical applications but also how, for example, the physicochemical properties of drugs such as their lipophilicity and aqueous solubility affect their pharmacokinetics, the relationships among Lipinski's rule of five, the biopharmaceutics classification system (BCS), and pharmacokinetics, and the pharmacokinetics of soft drugs and prodrugs. The pharmacokinetics of pharmaceutical excipients and how the excipients affect drug pharmacokinetics are also discussed. The text describes the effects of the routes of administration on drug pharmacokinetics. Numerous equations, practical examples, figures, and problems, with answers, have been included to facilitate self-study.

Chapter 1

Introduction

Chapter Outline

Although the concept of drug absorption, distribution and elimination has been known for over 150 years [1] the term "pharmacokinetics" was first introduced in 1953 by Friedrich Hartmut Dost in his book "Der Blütspiege: Kinetic der Konzentrationsabläufe in der Krieslaufflüssigkeit" [2,3]. Later Perl [4], Nelson [5], Krüger-Thiemer [6], Wagner [7,8], Garrett [9,10], Rowland [11], Gibaldi [12,13], Riegelman [14], Levy [15], and numerous other scientists introduced the various pharmacokinetic methods and terms, giving us the science of pharmacokinetics as it is today [1].

1.1 SOME BASIC CONCEPTS

A drug proceeds through a distinct pathway from mixing the active pharmaceutical ingredient (API) with excipients to forming the drug product to the therapeutic effect (Figure 1.1). For example, a propranolol tablet is formed by compressing a mixture of the API (i.e., propranolol hydrochloride) and various excipients such as lactose into a tablet. Tablets are one of several different propranolol drug products. Other known propranolol products include oral solutions and solutions for parenteral injection. Following oral administration (sometimes referred to as *per os* or *per oral* [PO] administration), the tablet disintegrates, and solid propranolol dissolves in the aqueous fluid of the gastrointestinal (GI) tract. The dissolved propranolol molecules are then absorbed into the general blood circulation and distributed throughout the body. The drug is partly metabolized and excreted from the body, but a small fraction of the drug, which is a β-blocker, reaches the target site, where its binds to receptors (e.g., β-adrenergic receptors), causing vasodilatation (which is the pharmacologic response) that leads to lowering of blood pressure (which is the therapeutic effect). *Pharmacokinetics* is the kinetics of

Essential Pharmacokinetics. DOI: http://dx.doi.org/10.1016/B978-0-12-801411-0.00001-9

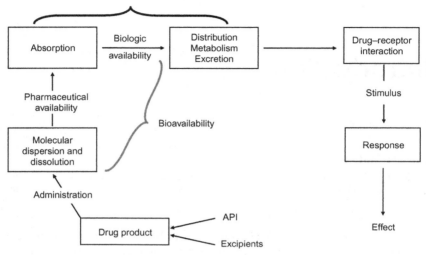

FIGURE 1.1   The drug pathway when, for example, administered orally.

drug absorption, distribution, metabolism, and excretion (ADME). All of these four criteria influence the levels and kinetics of drug exposure to tissues and thus influence the performance and pharmacologic activity of the compound as a drug. ADME profiling and toxicology screening are some of the most important research activities in the drug discovery and development process. ADME and toxicologic (ADME/Tox) properties determine the "druggability" of new chemical entities (NCEs). *Biopharmaceutics* describes how the physicochemical properties of drugs, the pharmaceutical dosage forms, and the routes of drug delivery affect the rate and extent of drug absorption into the body. *Pharmacodynamics* is the science that describes the relationship between the drug concentration at the receptor and biological activity (i.e., pharmacologic response or drug effect).

After oral administration, the drug is absorbed from the GI tract into the body (Figure 1.2). In general, some fraction of the drug is then metabolized and the metabolites excreted through urine, but a fraction of the drug may also be excreted unchanged through urine.

Bioavailability represents the drug fraction that reaches the systemic blood circulation after, for example, oral administration. Bioavailability can be divided into *pharmaceutical availability* and *biologic availability*. If propranolol is completely released from a tablet and dissolved in the aqueous GI fluid, the drug is said to have 100% pharmaceutical availability. Aqueous propranolol solution has 100% pharmaceutical availability (F_{pharm}). However, propranolol undergoes first-pass metabolism and thus its biologic availability (F_{bio}) after

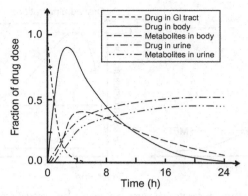

FIGURE 1.2 Schematic drawing showing the course of a drug and its metabolites after oral administration, expressed as a fraction of drug dose, within the body as intact drug and metabolites as well as in the GI tract and urine.

oral administration is frequently about 75%. Consequently, the bioavailability (F) of propranolol solution will be only about 75%:

$$F = F_{pharm} \times F_{bio} = 1.00 \times 0.75 = 0.75 \tag{1.1}$$

If the pharmaceutical availability of propranolol in a tablet is 50% and the biologic availability is 75%, the bioavailability of the propranolol tablets will be 37.5%:

$$F = F_{pharm} \times F_{bio} = 0.50 \times 0.75 = 0.375 \tag{1.2}$$

Drugs have 100% bioavailability when they are administered through intravenous (IV) injection, that is, the entire drug dose enters the general blood circulation. *Minimum effective concentration* (MEC) is the minimum plasma concentration of a drug needed to achieve sufficient drug concentration at the receptors to produce the desired pharmacologic response, if drug molecules in plasma are in equilibrium with drug molecules in the various tissues (Figure 1.3). *Minimum toxic concentration* (MTC) is the minimum drug plasma concentration that produces a toxic effect. *Onset time* is the time from administration that is required for a drug to reach its MEC. *Duration* of drug action is the difference between the onset time and the time when the drug concentration declines below MEC (Figure 1.3).

After oral administration, the drug is absorbed from the GI tract into the general blood circulation, where it reaches maximum plasma concentration (C_{max}) at time (t) equals t_{max}. Then the concentration declines as a result of metabolism and excretion of unmetabolized drug. The *therapeutic concentration range* (or *therapeutic window*) of a drug is the concentration range from the MEC to the MTC. In animal studies, the *therapeutic index* (TI) is the lethal dose of a drug for 50% of the animal population (LD_{50}) divided by the minimum effective dose for 50% of the population (ED_{50}). In humans, TI is

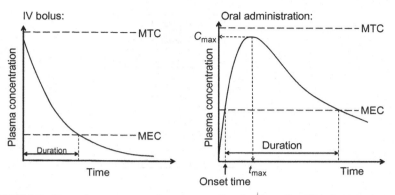

FIGURE 1.3 Drug plasma concentration−time profile of a drug after IV bolus injection and oral administration.

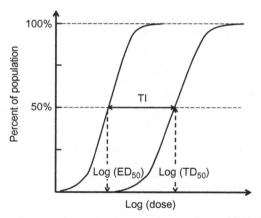

FIGURE 1.4 Drug dose−response relationship for producing the desired therapeutic effect and a toxic side effect (see section 5.3).

frequently defined as the ratio of the dose that produces toxicity in 50% of the population (TD_{50}) divided by ED_{50} (Figure 1.4):

$$\text{In animals:} \quad TI = \frac{LD_{50}}{ED_{50}} \tag{1.3}$$

$$\text{In humans:} \quad TI = \frac{TD_{50}}{ED_{50}} \tag{1.4}$$

1.2 PHARMACOKINETIC MODELS

Various types of pharmacokinetic models are used to describe drug absorption, distribution, metabolism, and elimination from the body (i.e., ADME). There are three basic types of pharmacokinetic modes: (1) *compartmental*

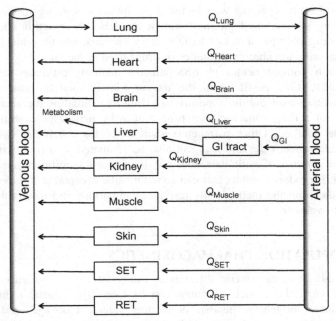

FIGURE 1.5 A physiologic-based pharmacokinetic model, in which compartments are used to represent different organs or group of tissues. Q is the rate of blood flow to the tissue, SETs are slowly equilibrating tissues, and RETs are the rapidly equilibrating tissues.

models, where a compartment represents a group of tissues that have similar affinity to the drug; (2) *physiologic-based pharmacokinetic models*, which apply physiologic parameters such as blood flow and drug partition into tissues; and (3) *noncompartmental models*, which use time and drug concentration averages. In compartmental models, groups of tissues that have similar blood flow and drug affinity are represented as single compartments. The compartments do not represent any specific anatomic region within the body. Uniform drug distribution is assumed within each compartment, and simple first-order rate equations are used to describe the transport of drug into and out of the compartment. Since the drug can enter and leave the body, the models are characterized as "open" models. The *caternary model*, in which the compartments are arranged like train wagons, and the *mammillary model*, which consists of one central compartment connected to peripheral compartments, are examples of compartmental pharmacokinetic models. The most common pharmacokinetic model in humans, and the only one discussed in this book, is the mammillary model.

Ideally, each and every tissue and body organ should be represented by one compartment, but the complexity of the human anatomy and physiology makes it virtually impossible. However, in physiologic-based pharmacokinetic models, some organs or tissues are represented by single compartments, whereas others are grouped into paired compartments (Figure 1.5). The blood flow (Q) to each organ, as well as the drug uptake to the organ, has to be known. Physiologic-based pharmacokinetic models are sometimes used to describe drug pharmacokinetics in laboratory animals, but they are seldom used to describe the pharmacokinetics of drugs used in humans.

Although compartmental pharmacokinetic methods estimate the drug concentration–time profile with the use of kinetic models, noncompartmental methods estimate the exposure to a drug by estimating the area under the curve of a drug concentration–time profile by using, for example, the trapezoidal method. Other parameters such as biologic half-life ($t_{1/2}$) of a drug, its clearance, C_{max} and t_{max} can also be estimated. Noncompartmental analysis of pharmacokinetic data does not assume any specific compartmental model. It produces results that can sometimes be acceptable in bioequivalence studies, but the method only provides estimations and results that are difficult to validate.

1.3 POPULATION PHARMACOKINETICS

Considerable pharmacokinetic differences can exist among patients (interindividual variability). Such variations can be caused by genetic influences, environmental influences, gender, drug–drug interactions, age, and body weight. Also, diseases can cause a patient to respond differently to a drug from 1 day to another (intraindividual variability). *Population pharmacokinetics* is the study of the sources of such variability. Population pharmacokinetics seeks to identify the measurable pathophysiologic factors such as kidney and liver functions that cause changes in the drug dose–concentration relationship and the extent of these changes so that dosage can be appropriately modified. Due to inter- and intraindividual variability, the administration of drugs with a narrow therapeutic concentration range needs to be individualized. *Therapeutic drug monitoring* (TDM) refers to individualization of drug dosage by maintaining drug plasma concentration within the therapeutic concentration range. Frequently, such monitoring is based on clinical observations and determination of drug plasma concentrations. Therapeutic concentration ranges of selected drugs are displayed in Table 1.1.

Pharmacokinetics is used to optimize the administration and the therapeutic effects of drugs, as well as the design and evaluation of drug dosage forms. For example, pharmacokinetics can be used to:

1. Calculate loading and maintenance drug doses. The *loading dose* is a large initial dose given to achieve therapeutic drug levels from the beginning; a *maintenance dose* is then given at fixed intervals to keep drug concentrations within the therapeutic range.
2. Calculate drug dosage regimen. The dosage regimen is a systemized dosage schedule with two variables: (a) the size of each drug dose and (b) the time between consecutive dose administrations. Dosage regimen

TABLE 1.1 Therapeutic Concentration Ranges of Some Selected Drugs in Plasma

Drug	Therapeutic usage	Therapeutic concentration range (μg/ml)
Amiodarone	Antiarrhythmic agent	1.0−2.5
Amitriptyline	Tricyclic antidepressant	0.12−0.15
Carbamazepine	Anticonvulsant	4−12
Cyclosporine	Immunosuppressant	0.15−0.40
Digoxin	Cardiac glycoside	0.0006−0.002
Gentamycin	Aminoglycoside antibiotic	4−12
Lidocaine	Local anesthetic and antiarrhythmic drug	1.5−5.0
Nortriptyline	Tricyclic antidepressant	0.05−0.15
Phenobarbitone	Anticonvulsant	15−40
Salicylate	Nonsteroidal anti-inflammatory drug	50−250
Theophylline	Antiasthmatic drug, bronchodilator	10−20
Valproic acid	Anticonvulsant	40−100
Vancomycin	Glycopeptide antibiotic	20−40
Warfarin	Anticoagulant	1−4

calculations are frequently based on population pharmacokinetics and therapeutic drug monitoring.

3. Perform dosage adjustments in patients with, for example, renal and hepatic diseases.
4. Design of dosage form and determination of route of administration, for example, sustained-release versus immediate-release oral dosage forms, and parenteral versus oral dosage forms. The route of administration can affect drug pharmacokinetics.
5. Perform bioequivalence studies, that is, pharmacokinetic evaluations of drug formulations. Some pharmaceutical excipients can enhance or decrease drug bioavailability.
6. Predict drug−drug and drug−food interactions. Both co-administered drugs and various food products can interfere with drug absorption, distribution, metabolism, and excretion.

REFERENCES

[1]   Wagner JG. History of pharmacokinetics. Pharmac Ther 1981;12:537–62.

[2]   Dost FH. Der Blutspiegel: Kinetik der Kozentrationsabläufe in der Kreislaufflüssigkeit. Leipzig: G. Thieme; 1953.

[3]   Dost FH. Grundlagen der pharmakokinetik. Stuttgart: G. Thieme; 1968.

[4]   Perl W, Lesser GT, Steele JM. The kinetics of distribution of the fat-soluble inert gas cyclopropane in the body. Biophys J 1960;1:111–35.

[5]   Nelson E. Kinetics of drug absorption, distribution, metabolism and excretion. J Pharm Sci 1961;50:181–92.

[6]   Krüger-Thiemer E. Dosage schedules and pharmacokinetics in chemotherapy. J Am Pharm Assoc Sci Ed 1960;49:311–13.

[7]   Wagner JG. Fundamentals of clinical pharmacokinetics. Hamilton: Drug Intelligence Publications; 1975.

[8]   Wagner JG. Pharmacokinetics for the pharmaceutical scientist. Technomic Publishing Co., Basel; 1993.

[9]   Garrett ER. Physicochemical and pharmacokinetic bases for the biopharmaceutical evaluation of drug biological availability in pharmaceutical formulations. Acta Pharmacol Toxicol (Copenh) 1971;(Suppl.23):1–29.

[10] Garrett ER. Basic concepts and experimental methods of pharmacokinetics. Adv Biosci 1970;5:7–20.

[11] Rowland M, Benet LZ, Graham CG. Clearance concepts in pharmacokinetics. J Pharmacok Biopharm 1973;1:123–36.

[12] Gibaldi M, Perrier D. Pharmacokinetics. New York, NY: Marcel Dekker; 1975.

[13] Gibaldi M. Biopharmaceutics and clinical pharmacokinetics. Philadelphia, PA: Lea and Febiger; 1977.

[14] Riegelman S. Physiological and pharmacokinetic complexities in bioavailability testing. Pharmacology 1972;8:118–41.

[15] Levy G. Kinetics of drug action: an overview. J Allergy Clin Immunol 1986;78:754–61.

Chapter 2

Basic Concepts of Pharmacokinetics

Chapter Outline

The mammillary model is the most common pharmacokinetic model. It is an empirical model that does not explain the actual mechanisms by which the drug is absorbed, distributed, and eliminated from the body. The mammillary

Essential Pharmacokinetics. DOI: http://dx.doi.org/10.1016/B978-0-12-801411-0.00002-0

model is a compartmental model, in which groups of tissues that have similar blood flow and drug affinity are represented by a single compartment. Thus, a compartment is not a real anatomic region within the body. Uniform drug distribution is assumed within each compartment, and simple first-order rate equations are used to describe transport of drug into and out of the compartment. Since the drug can enter and leave the body, the model is characterized as an "open" model.

2.1 ONE-COMPARTMENT OPEN MODEL

The one-compartment open model is the simplest mammillary model that describes drug distribution and elimination. In the one-compartment model, the body is described as a single, uniform compartment into which the drug is administered and from which it is eliminated. This is a very simplistic view of the body, in which the drug enters the bloodstream and is then rapidly equilibrated with other parts of the body. This model does not predict actual drug concentrations in the various tissues but assumes that drug tissue concentrations will be proportional to the drug plasma concentrations.

2.1.1 IV Bolus Injection

In the one-compartment open model, after IV bolus administration, the entire drug dose enters the blood circulation immediately and is then distributed very rapidly throughout the body (Figure 2.1). The drug equilibrates rapidly in the body, and it is assumed that the concentration throughout the compartment is equal to the plasma concentration (C_P). The *elimination rate constant* (k) is composed of the first-order rate constant for the drug metabolism (k_m) and the first-order rate constant for the renal excretion (k_e) of unmetabolized drug or $k = k_m + k_e$. The dose is the amount of drug in the body at time (t) = 0 or D_0.

The drug elimination from the body follows simple first-order kinetics:

$$\frac{dD_B}{dt} = -k \cdot D_B \tag{2.1}$$

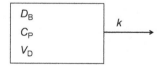

FIGURE 2.1 One-compartment open model. The drug is administered via rapid IV injection and is rapidly distributed throughout the body. The drug molecules in plasma are in a dynamic equilibrium with drug molecules in the various body tissues. D_B, Total amount of drug in the body; C_P, plasma concentration of the drug; V_D, apparent volume of distribution; k, first-order elimination rate constant.

where D_B is the total amount of drug within the body. Integration of Eq. (2.1) gives Eqs. (2.2) and (2.3):

$$\ln D_B = \ln D_B - k \cdot t \qquad (2.2)$$

$$D_B = D_0 \cdot e^{-k \cdot t} \qquad (2.3)$$

At $t = 0$, no drug has been excreted from the body; that is, the entire drug dose is located in the compartment (D_B at time 0 is equal to D_0). Thus, the *apparent volume of distribution* (V_D) is equal to D_0 divided by the drug plasma concentration at $t = 0$ (C_P^0):

$$V_D = \frac{D_0}{C_P^0} \qquad (2.4)$$

V_D is the volume of the theoretical compartment, which can be smaller or larger than the actual volume of the body. Combining Eqs. (2.2) and (2.4) and Eqs. (2.3) and (2.4) gives Eqs. (2.5) and (2.6), respectively:

$$C_P = \frac{D_0}{V_D} \cdot e^{-k \cdot t} \qquad (2.5)$$

$$\ln C_P = \ln C_P^0 - k \cdot t \qquad (2.6)$$

The biologic half-life ($t_{1/2}$) of a drug that follows first-order elimination kinetics, that is, the half-life of drug elimination from the body, is independent of the total amount of the drug in the body:

$$t_{1/2} = \frac{\ln 2}{k} \qquad (2.7)$$

Clearance (drug clearance) is a measure of drug elimination from the body without identifying the mechanism or process. Strictly speaking, clearance is the volume of plasma cleared of the drug per unit time. Clearance can be divided into total body clearance (Cl_T), renal clearance (Cl_R), hepatic clearance (Cl_H), and so on:

$$Cl_T = V_D \cdot k \qquad (2.8)$$

$$Cl_T = Cl_R + Cl_H + \cdots = V_D \cdot k_e + V_D \cdot k_m + \cdots \qquad (2.9)$$

$$Cl_T = Cl_R + Cl_{NR} \qquad (2.10)$$

where Cl_{NR} is the non-renal clearance, including Cl_H. The area under the plasma concentration−time curve (AUC) from time zero to infinity (∞) is obtained by integrating Eq. (2.3) from $t = 0$ to $t = \infty$ giving Eq. (2.12):

$$\int_0^{D_0} dD_0 = -k \cdot V_D \cdot \int_0^{\infty} C_p dt \qquad (2.11)$$

$$[AUC]_0^\infty = \frac{D_0}{V_D \cdot k} \tag{2.12}$$

Rearrangement of Eq. (2.12) gives Eqs. (2.13) and (2.14):

$$V_D = \frac{D_0}{[AUC]_0^\infty \cdot k} \tag{2.13}$$

$$Cl_T = k \cdot V_D = \frac{D_0}{[AUC]_0^\infty} \tag{2.14}$$

The area under the curve (AUC) can be estimated graphically (e.g., by the trapezoidal method), and the AUC thus obtained can be inserted into Eq. (2.13) to calculate V_D. Consequently, Eq. (2.13) is said to be a model-independent method for calculation of V_D.

It should be emphasized that in the mammillary model, V_D is generally not a real volume but an apparent volume determined by assuming that the drug concentration throughout the body is the same as in plasma. In an average adult person, the plasma volume is 2.7–3.0 liters or approximately 0.04 l/kg. Drugs with V_D greater than 0.04 l/kg are distributed outside plasma, but the actual size of the distribution volume cannot be determined from the V_D value. V_D can be much larger than the body volume (Table 2.1). Lipophilic drugs tend to have larger V_D than hydrophilic drugs. Drugs that are highly bound to proteins in plasma tend to have smaller V_D than drugs displaying less protein binding.

TABLE 2.1 Examples of Volume of Distribution (V_D) and Half-Lives ($t_{1/2}$). In Normal Individuals the Volume of Plasma is Approximately 0.04 l/kg

Drug	V_D (l/kg)	$t_{1/2}$ (h)
Amoxicillin	0.21	1.7
Aspirin	0.15	0.25
Diazepam	1.1	43
Enalapril	1.7	11
2-Hydroxypropyl-β-cyclodextrin	0.2	0.4
Ibuprofen	0.15	2.0
Nitroglycerin	3.3	0.04
Warfarin	0.14	37

EXAMPLE 2.1 Salicylic Acid—IV Bolus, One-Compartment Model

A 65 kg man was given a single 600 mg IV bolus dose of salicylic acid ($D_0 = 600$ mg). Blood samples were taken at various time intervals and the plasma concentration of the drug (C_P) determined:

Time (h)	C_P (μg/ml)
1	42.0
2	33.0
3	28.0
4	22.5
6	14.5

Calculate the plasma concentration at time zero (C_P^0), the apparent volume of distribution (V_D), the elimination rate constant (k), the biologic half-life of the drug ($t_{1/2}$), the drug plasma concentration 20 hours after its administration (C_P^{20}), and the total body clearance (Cl_T). What is the renal clearance (Cl_R) if 25% of salicylic acid is excreted unchanged with the urine?

Answer
Plot the results according to Eq. (2.6).

Time (h)	ln C_P
1	3.74
2	3.50
3	3.33
4	3.11
6	2.67

C_P^0 cannot be determined directly but has to be estimated from the y-intercept, as shown in Figure 2.2:

$$\ln C_P^0 = 3.9468 \Rightarrow C_P^0 = 51.8 \ \mu\text{g/ml}$$

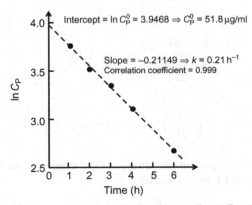

FIGURE 2.2 Plot of ln C_P versus time for salicylic acid according to Eq. (2.6).

The elimination rate constant is determined from the slope (Figure 2.2): $k = 0.21\ \mathrm{h}^{-1}$. Then, V_D, $t_{1/2}$, C_P^{20}, Cl_T, and Cl_R are determined:

$$V_D = \frac{D_0}{C_P^0} = \frac{600\ \mathrm{mg}}{51.8\ \mathrm{mg/l}} = 11.6\ \mathrm{l}$$

$$t_{1/2} = \frac{\ln 2}{k} = \frac{0.693}{0.21\ \mathrm{h}^{-1}} = 3.3\ \mathrm{h}$$

$$C_P^{20} = \frac{D_0}{V_D} \cdot e^{-k \cdot t} = \frac{600\ \mathrm{mg}}{11.6\ \mathrm{l}} \cdot e^{-0.21 \cdot 20} = 0.78\ \mathrm{mg/l} = 0.78\ \mathrm{\mu g/ml}$$

$Cl_T = V_D \cdot k = 11.6\ \mathrm{l} \cdot 0.21\ \mathrm{h}^{-1} = 2.4\ \mathrm{l/h} = 41\ \mathrm{ml/min}$ or $Cl_T = \frac{41\ \mathrm{ml/min}}{65\ \mathrm{kg}} = 0.63\ \mathrm{ml/min \cdot kg}$

$$Cl_R = 0.25 \cdot Cl_T = 0.25 \cdot 41 = 10\ \mathrm{ml/min}\ \text{or}\ 0.16\ \mathrm{ml/min \cdot kg}$$

The elimination rate constant (k) may also be calculated from the urinary excretion data and even from the excretion data of drugs by other body fluids such as saliva. k is composed of the first-order renal excretion rate constant (k_e), the first-order rate constant for metabolism (k_m), the first-order rate constant for biliary excretion (k_b), and so on:

$$k = k_e + k_m + k_b + \cdots \tag{2.15}$$

$$k_e = k - (k_m + k_b + \cdots) = k - k_{nr} \tag{2.16}$$

where k_{nr} is the sum of all the other rate constants except k_e (i.e., $k_{nr} = k_m + k_b + \cdots$). The rate of elimination of unmetabolized drug with urine follows first-order kinetics:

$$\frac{dD_U}{dt} = k_e \cdot D_B \tag{2.17}$$

Combining Eqs. (2.3) and (2.17) gives:

$$\frac{dD_U}{dt} = k_e \cdot D_0 \cdot e^{-k \cdot t} \tag{2.18}$$

$$\ln\left(\frac{dD_U}{dt}\right) = \ln(k_e \cdot D_0) - k \cdot t \tag{2.19}$$

Equation (2.19) is an equation of a straight line, where k_e can be determined from the intercept and k from the slope.

EXAMPLE 2.2 Urinary Excretion Data—IV Bolus, One-Compartment Model

A digitalis glycoside (0.6 mg) was administered via IV bolus injection and the amount excreted unchanged with urine determined:

Time (days)	Urine volume (ml)	Drug urinary concentration (ng/ml)
0–1	1,000	139
1–2	1,100	89
2–3	1,300	52
3–5	2,500	35

Calculate $t_{1/2}$, k, k_e, and k_{nr}. How large is the fraction of the drug that is excreted unchanged with the urine?

Answer

Plot the data according to Eq. (2.19), where t_m is the midpoint of urine collection (Figure 2.3):

$$\ln\left(\frac{\Delta D_U}{\Delta t}\right) = \ln(k_e \cdot D_0) - k \cdot t_m$$

Time (days)	V_U (ml)	C_U (ng/ml)	ΔD_U (μg)	Δt (days)	$\Delta D_U/\Delta t$ (μg/days)	t_m (days)	$\ln(\Delta D_U/\Delta t)$
0–1	1,000	139	139.0	1	139.0	0.5	4.934
1–2	1,100	89	97.9	1	97.9	1.5	4.584
2–3	1,300	53	68.9	1	68.9	2.5	4.233
3–5	2,500	34	85.0	2	42.5	4.0	3.750

$$k = 0.362 \text{ days}^{-1} \text{ and } t_{1/2} = \frac{\ln 2}{k} = \frac{0.693}{0.362 \text{ days}^{-1}} = 1.91 \text{ days}$$

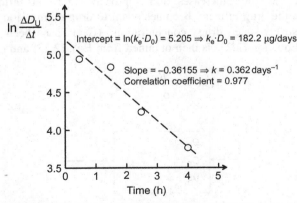

FIGURE 2.3   Plot of $\ln(\Delta D_U/\Delta t)$ versus time according to Eq. (2.19).

$$\ln(k_e D_0) = 5.205 \Rightarrow k_e \cdot D_0 = 182.18 \ \mu g/\text{days} \Rightarrow k_e = \frac{182.18 \ \mu g/\text{days}^{-1}}{D_0}$$

$$= \frac{182.18 \ \mu g/\text{days}^{-1}}{600 \ \mu g} = 0.30 \ \text{days}^{-1}$$

Fraction excreted unchanged with urine:

$$f_e = \frac{k_e}{k} = \frac{0.30 \ \text{days}^{-1}}{0.362 \ \text{days}^{-1}} = 0.83 \quad \text{or} \quad 83\%$$

2.1.2 IV Infusion

When a drug follows a one-compartment model, after slow IV infusion, the drug is distributed very rapidly throughout the body after it enters the general blood circulation (Figure 2.4). The infusion rate (R) is zero order but the elimination rate constant (k) is as before first order.

The change in the amount of drug in the body (dD_B/dt) will be:

$$\frac{dD_B}{dt} = R - k \cdot D_B \tag{2.20}$$

where R is the infusion rate (zero-order rate constant). Integration of Eq. (2.20) gives:

$$D_B = \frac{R}{k} \cdot (1 - e^{-k \cdot t}) \tag{2.21}$$

Combining $D_B = C_P \cdot V_D$ and Eq. (2.21) gives:

$$C_P = \frac{R}{V_D \cdot k} \cdot (1 - e^{-k \cdot t}) \tag{2.22}$$

$e^{-k \cdot t}$ decreases as time increases and approaches zero at infinite time ($t = \infty$). Then the drug infusion becomes equal to drug elimination from the body, and steady-state drug concentration (C_{SS}) has been reached (Figure 2.5). Equation (2.23) is then obtained from Eqs. (2.22) and (2.8):

$$C_{SS} = \frac{R}{V_D \cdot k} = \frac{R}{Cl_T} \tag{2.23}$$

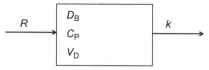

FIGURE 2.4 One-compartment open model where the drug is administered by IV infusion and is rapidly distributed throughout the body. R is the zero-order drug infusion rate constant.

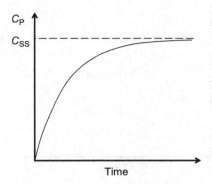

FIGURE 2.5   Plot of C_P versus time for according to Eq. (2.22). The steady-state drug concentration (C_{SS}) is obtained when $t = \infty$.

How long does it take to reach 50%, 90%, 99%, and 99.9% of C_{SS} after IV infusion has started?

$$C_P = \frac{R}{V_D \cdot k} \cdot (1 - e^{-k \cdot t}) = C_{SS} \cdot (1 - e^{-k \cdot t}) \Rightarrow \frac{C_P}{C_{SS}} = (1 - e^{-k \cdot t})$$

50% of C_{SS}: $0.50 = (1 - e^{-k \cdot t}) \Rightarrow 0.50 = e^{-k \cdot t} \Rightarrow -k \cdot t = -0.693$ or $t = \frac{0.693}{k} = t_{1/2}$.
Thus, it takes one half-life ($t_{1/2}$) to reach 50% of C_{SS}.
90% of C_{SS}: $0.90 = (1 - e^{-k \cdot t}) \Rightarrow 0.10 = e^{-k \cdot t} \Rightarrow -k \cdot t = -2.3026$ or $t = 3.32 \cdot t_{1/2}$.
99% of C_{SS}: $0.99 = (1 - e^{-k \cdot t}) \Rightarrow 0.01 = e^{-k \cdot t} \Rightarrow -k \cdot t = -4.6052$ or $t = 6.64 \cdot t_{1/2}$.
99.9% of C_{SS}: $0.999 = (1 - e^{-k \cdot t}) \Rightarrow 0.001 = e^{-k \cdot t} \Rightarrow -k \cdot t = -6.9078$ or $t = 9.97 \cdot t_{1/2}$.
It takes indefinite time ($t = \infty$) to reach C_{SS} but 10 half-lives to reach 99.9% of C_{SS}.

A *loading dose* (D_L) can be given as an IV bolus dose to obtain the target drug plasma concentration, that is, C_{SS}, at the start of drug infusion:

$$D_L = V_D \cdot C_{SS} \qquad (2.24)$$

The total drug plasma concentration will then be the sum of the loading dose given via IV bolus injection that follows first-order elimination kinetics and the maintenance dose given as IV infusion (R) that follows zero-order drug delivery and first-order drug elimination kinetics (Eq. (2.25) and Figure 2.6):

$$C_P = \frac{D_L}{V_D} \cdot e^{-k \cdot t} + \frac{R}{V_D \cdot k} \cdot (1 - e^{-k \cdot t}) = C_{SS} \qquad (2.25)$$

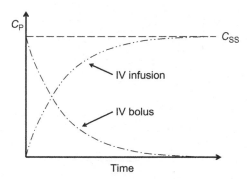

FIGURE 2.6 Intravenous infusion with a loading dose (D_L) given as IV bolus injection at the start of drug infusion. The sum of the loading dose and the infusion gives a straight line representing C_{SS} (Eqs. (2.25) and (2.27)).

By combining Eqs. (2.23) and (2.24), we get:

$$D_L = \frac{R}{k} \qquad (2.26)$$

Combining Eqs. (2.23) and (2.25) gives:

$$C_P = C_{SS} = \frac{R}{V_D \cdot k} \qquad (2.27)$$

EXAMPLE 2.3   IV Infusion and a Loading Dose

An antibiotic ($t_{\frac{1}{2}} = 2.6$ h, $V_D = 20$ L) is given via IV infusion. Therapeutic plasma concentration is 6 µg/ml, and the drug concentration of the parenteral solution is 1 mg/ml. Determine the infusion rate constant. How long does it take C_P to reach 99% of C_{SS}? Calculate D_L that gives $C_P = C_{SS}$ from the beginning of drug infusion.

Answer

$$C_{SS} = \frac{R}{V_D \cdot k} = \frac{R \cdot t_{\frac{1}{2}}}{V_D \cdot 0.693} \Rightarrow R = \frac{C_{SS} \cdot V_D \cdot \ln 2}{t_{\frac{1}{2}}} = \frac{6 \text{ mg/l} \cdot 20 \text{ l} \cdot 0.693}{2.6 \text{ h}}$$

$$= 32 \text{ mg/h} \text{ or } R = 32 \text{ ml/h}$$

99% of C_{SS}: $t_{99\%} = 6.64 \cdot t_{\frac{1}{2}} = 6.64 \cdot 2.6 \text{ h} = 17 \text{ h}$

$$D_L = \frac{R}{k} = C_{SS} \cdot V_D = 6 \text{ mg/l} \cdot 20 \text{ l} = 120 \text{ mg}$$

EXAMPLE 2.4   IV Infusion Discontinued

The drug in Example 2.3 was given as an infusion for 12 h without a loading dose. What is the concentration 6 h after the infusion was stopped (Figure 2.7)?

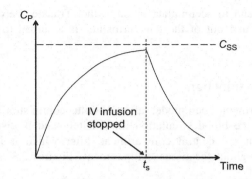

FIGURE 2.7 C_P–time profile after IV infusion that is stopped at $t = t_s$ with a first-order C_P decline.

Answer

At 12 h: $\frac{C_P}{C_{SS}} = (1 - e^{-k \cdot t}) = (1 - e^{-(\ln 2/2.6 \text{ h}) \cdot 12 \text{ h}}) = 0.959$ or C_P is 95.9% of C_{SS}

You can solve this problem by using Eq. (2.22) to calculate C_P at 12 h and then Eq. (2.5) to calculate C_P 6 h after infusion was stopped or you can combine Eqs. (2.5) and (2.22) and use that new equation to calculate C_P in one step:

$$C_P = \frac{R}{V_D \cdot k} \cdot (1 - e^{-k \cdot t_s}) \cdot e^{-k \cdot (t - t_s)} \qquad (2.28)$$

where t_s is the time when infusion was stopped (here 12 h) and t is the total time, that is, infusion time and post-infusion time (here 18 h):

$$C_P^{18} = \frac{32 \text{ mg/h}}{20 \text{ L} \cdot (\ln 2/2.6 \text{ h})} \cdot (1 - e^{-(\ln 2/2.6 \text{ h}) \cdot 12 \text{ h}}) \cdot e^{-(\ln 2/2.6 \text{ h}) \cdot (18 - 12) \text{ h}}$$

$$= 6.000 \text{ mg/l} \cdot 0.959 \cdot 0.2019 = 1.16 \text{ mg/l} \quad \text{or} \quad C_P^{18} = 1.16 \text{ μg/ml}$$

2.2   TWO-COMPARTMENT OPEN MODEL

In the two-compartment open model, the body is described as two hypothetical compartments: (1) the *central compartment*, which represents blood, extracellular fluid, and highly perfused tissues, and (2) *tissue compartment* (sometimes called the *peripheral compartment*), which contains tissues such as skin and fat tissue, in which the drug equilibrates more slowly. The heart, liver, kidneys, lungs, and brain are highly perfused organs, which generally belong to the central compartment. The drug enters the body and leaves it via the central compartment. This model does not predict actual drug concentrations in various tissues but assumes that drug tissue concentrations are uniform throughout the compartment. Distribution of a given drug within a compartment will, however, depend on its physicochemical properties. Highly protein-bound drugs tend to be concentrated in plasma, whereas lipophilic drugs tend to accumulate in fat tissue. Transfer between the two compartments, in and out of the compartments, is assumed to follow first-order kinetics.

2.2.1 IV Bolus Injection

In the two-compartment open model, after IV bolus administration, the entire drug dose enters the blood circulation immediately and is distributed very rapidly throughout the central compartment, after which it is distributed more slowly throughout the tissue compartment (Figures 2.8 and 2.9). The

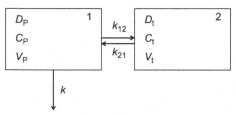

FIGURE 2.8 Two-compartment open model. The drug is administered by rapid IV injection into the central compartment (compartment 1), where it is rapidly distributed and reaches equilibrium. Then, it partitions into the tissue compartment (compartment 2), where it is more slowly equilibrated. D_P, amount of drug in central compartment; C_P, plasma concentration of the drug; V_P, apparent volume of central compartment (volume of plasma); D_t, amount of drug in tissue compartment; C_t, hypothetical drug tissue concentration; V_t, apparent volume of tissue compartment; k, overall first-order elimination rate constant; k_{12}, transfer rate constant from compartment 1 to compartment 2; k_{21} = transfer rate constant from compartment 2 to compartment 1.

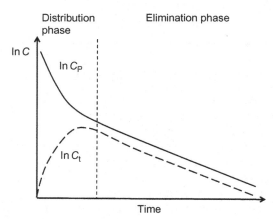

FIGURE 2.9 Plasma (*solid curve*) and tissue (*dashed curve*) drug concentration−time curves for a drug that follows the two-compartment open model after IV bolus injection. The tissue concentration (C_t) may be higher or lower than the plasma concentration (C_P). Here, the tissue concentration is lower than the plasma concentration.

drug is also excreted from the body via the central compartment, since the kidneys and liver are highly perfused organs that belong to the central compartment.

In the distribution phase (Figure 2.9), the plasma drug concentration falls rapidly due to simultaneous elimination and distribution into the tissue compartment. This is followed by much slower plasma drug concentration decline after equilibration between the central compartment and the tissue compartment has been reached in the elimination phase. Changes in C_P (i.e., drug concentration in the central compartment) and C_t (i.e., drug concentration in the tissue compartment) follow simple first-order kinetics:

$$\frac{dD_P}{dt} = k_{21} \cdot D_t - k_{12} \cdot D_P - k \cdot D_P \tag{2.29}$$

$$\frac{dD_t}{dt} = k_{12} \cdot D_P - k_{21} \cdot D_t \tag{2.30}$$

The drug concentration in each compartment is:

$$C_P = \frac{D_P}{V_P} \tag{2.31}$$

$$C_t = \frac{D_t}{V_t} \tag{2.32}$$

Combining the equations gives:

$$\frac{dC_P}{dt} = k_{21} \cdot \frac{D_t}{V_t} - k_{12} \cdot \frac{D_P}{V_P} - k \cdot \frac{D_P}{V_P} \tag{2.33}$$

$$\frac{dC_t}{dt} = k_{12} \cdot \frac{D_P}{V_P} - k_{21} \cdot \frac{D_t}{V_t} \tag{2.34}$$

Further manipulation of the equations gives the classic equation for drug distribution according to the two-compartment model after IV bolus injection:

$$C_P = Ae^{-a \cdot t} + Be^{-b \cdot t} \tag{2.35}$$

where a and b are first-order rate constants for the distribution phase and elimination phase, respectively, and A and B are the y-axis intercepts for the each of the two exponential functions. The constants A, B, a, and b may be obtained graphically or by fitting experimental drug plasma concentration−time data to Eq. (2.35). k, k_{12}, and k_{21} cannot be determined directly but can be estimated from the following equations:

$$a + b = k_{12} + k_{21} + k \tag{2.36}$$

$$a \cdot b = k_{21} \cdot k \tag{2.37}$$

$$k = \frac{a \cdot b \cdot (A + B)}{A \cdot b + B \cdot a} \tag{2.38}$$

$$k_{12} = \frac{A \cdot B \cdot (b-a)^2}{(A + B) \cdot (A \cdot b + B \cdot a)} \tag{2.39}$$

$$k_{21} = \frac{A \cdot b + B \cdot a}{A + B} \tag{2.40}$$

The rate constant b can be determined from the slope of the elimination phase and the half-life of the elimination phase (sometimes referred to as the beta half-life, $t_{\frac{1}{2}\beta}$ or $t_{\frac{1}{2}b}$) can be obtained from the rate constant:

$$t_{\frac{1}{2}b} = \frac{\ln 2}{b} = \frac{0.693}{b} \tag{2.41}$$

The volume of the central compartment (V_P) is calculated from the drug does (D_0) administered by IV bolus injection and the drug plasma concentration at $t = 0$ (C_P^0). According to Eq. (2.35):

$$C_P^0 = A + B \tag{2.42}$$

and

$$V_P = \frac{D_0}{A + B} \tag{2.43}$$

It is also possible to determine V_P from the AUC from time zero to infinity ($[AUC]_0^\infty$):

$$V_P = \frac{D_0}{k \cdot [AUC]_0^\infty} \tag{2.44}$$

V_P is used to calculate the drug clearance:

$$Cl_T = k \cdot V_P = \frac{D_0}{[AUC]_0^\infty} \tag{2.45}$$

Other types of volume of distribution in the two-compartment model include volume of distribution by area ($(V_D)_{area}$), extrapolated volume of distribution ($(V_D)_{exp}$), volume of distribution at steady-state ($(V_D)_{ss}$), and the apparent volume of the tissue compartment (V_t):

$$(V_D)_{area} = \frac{D_0}{b \cdot [AUC]_0^\infty} \tag{2.46}$$

$$Cl_T = b \cdot (V_D)_{area} = \frac{D_0}{[AUC]_0^\infty} \tag{2.47}$$

$$(V_D)_{exp} = \frac{D_0}{B} \tag{2.48}$$

$$(V_D)_{ss} = \frac{D_P + D_t}{C_P} = V_P + \frac{k_{12}}{k_{21}} \cdot V_P \tag{2.49}$$

$$V_t = \frac{k_{12}}{k_{21}} \cdot V_P \tag{2.50}$$

Integration of Eq. (2.35) from time 0 to ∞ gives:

$$[AUC]_0^\infty = \frac{A}{a} + \frac{B}{b} \tag{2.51}$$

EXAMPLE 2.5 IV Bolus and Two-Compartment Open Model

A 70 kg man was given a single 100 mg IV bolus dose of a drug ($D_0 = 100$ mg). Blood samples were collected and the plasma concentration of the drug (C_P) determined:

Time (min)	C_P (μg/ml)
5	2.07
10	1.60
15	1.28
30	0.80
60	0.53
90	0.41
120	0.33
180	0.21
240	0.13

Calculate A, B, a, b, k, k_{12}, k_{21}, $t_{1/2}$, V_P, $(V_D)_{area}$, V_t, and Cl_T.

Answer

First, the C_P versus time data are plotted. Below is a semilog plot with linear x-axis and logarithmic y-axis showing the two phases. The plot indicates that the drug follows the two-compartment model after IV bolus injection. It is sometimes difficult to distinguish between two- and three-compartment models, but three-compartment models are relatively rare. Thus, it is common to assume the two-compartment model when a semilog plot displays two phases. In rare cases, when a drug follows the three-compartment model, the third phase will be observed during extraction of the rate constants from the experimental plasma concentration–time data. The first exponent of Eq. (2.35) decreases much faster than the second exponent, and thus the first exponent in Eq. (2.35) can be ignored in the elimination phase:

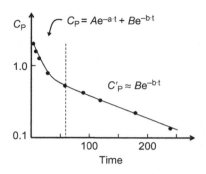

Time (min)	C_P (µg/ml)	ln C_P	C'_P (µg/ml)	$(C_P - C'_P)$ (µg/ml)	$ln(C_P - C'_P)$
5	2.07	0.728	0.803	1.27	0.237
10	1.60	0.470	0.772	0.828	−0.189
15	1.28	0.247	0.743	0.537	−0.622
30	0.80	−0.223	0.662	0.138	−1.978
60	0.53	−0.635			
90	0.41	−0.892			
120	0.33	−1.109			
180	0.21	−1.561			
240	0.13	−2.040			

$C_P = Ae^{-a \cdot t} + Be^{-b \cdot t}$

$ln(C_P - C'_P) = \ln A - a \cdot t$

$\ln C'_P = \ln B - b \cdot t$

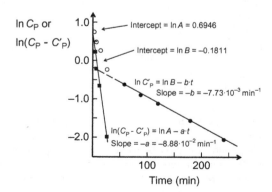

From the graph, it can be calculated that:

$A = 2.00$ µg/ml; $B = 0.83$ µg/ml; $a = 8.88 \cdot 10^{-2}$ min^{-1}; $b = 7.73 \cdot 10^{-3}$ min^{-1}

$C_P = 2.00 \cdot e^{-8.88 \cdot 10^{-2} \cdot t} + 0.83 \cdot e^{-7.73 \cdot 10^{-3} \cdot t}$ where C_P is in µg/ml and t in minutes.

Then, k, k_{12}, k_{21}, $t_{\frac{1}{2}}$, V_P, $(V_D)_{area}$, V_t, and Cl_T can be calculated:

$$k = \frac{a \cdot b \cdot (A+B)}{A \cdot b + B \cdot a} = \frac{8.88 \cdot 10^{-2} \cdot 7.73 \cdot 10^{-3} \cdot (2.00+0.83)}{2.00 \cdot 7.73 \cdot 10^{-3} + 0.83 \cdot 8.88 \cdot 10^{-2}} = 2.18 \cdot 10^{-2} \, min^{-1}$$

$$k_{12} = \frac{A \cdot B \cdot (b-a)^2}{(A+B) \cdot (A \cdot b + B \cdot a)} = \frac{2.00 \cdot 0.83 \cdot (7.73 \cdot 10^{-3} - 8.88 \cdot 10^{-2})^2}{(2.00+0.83) \cdot (2.00 \cdot 7.73 \cdot 10^{-3} + 0.83 \cdot 8.88 \cdot 10^{-2})}$$
$$= 4.32 \cdot 10^{-2} \, min^{-1}$$

$$k_{21} = \frac{A \cdot b + B \cdot a}{A+B} = \frac{2.00 \cdot 7.73 \cdot 10^{-3} + 0.83 \cdot 8.88 \cdot 10^{-2}}{2.00+0.83} = 3.15 \cdot 10^{-2} \, min^{-1}$$

We can use the following two equations to check the results:

$$a + b = k_{12} + k_{21} + k \Rightarrow 8.88 \cdot 10^{-2} + 7.73 \cdot 10^{-3} = 4.32 \cdot 10^{-2} + 3.15 \cdot 10^{-2}$$
$$+ 2.18 \cdot 10^{-2} \Rightarrow 9.65 \cdot 10^{-2} = 9.65 \cdot 10^{-2}$$

$$a \cdot b = k_{21} \cdot k \Rightarrow 8.88 \cdot 10^{-2} \cdot 7.73 \cdot 10^{-3} = 3.15 \cdot 10^{-2} \cdot 2.18 \cdot 10^{-2}$$
$$\Rightarrow 6.864 \cdot 10^{-4} \approx 6.867 \cdot 10^{-4}$$

Then, we calculate the other parameters:

$$t_{\frac{1}{2}} = \frac{\ln 2}{b} = \frac{0.693}{b} = \frac{0.693}{7.73 \cdot 10^{-3}} = 90 \, min$$

$$V_P = \frac{D_0}{A+B} = \frac{100 \, mg}{(2.00+0.83) mg/l} = 35.3 \, l$$

$$[AUC]_0^\infty = \frac{A}{a} + \frac{B}{b} = \frac{2.00}{8.88 \cdot 10^{-2}} + \frac{0.83}{7.73 \cdot 10^{-3}} = 130 \, mg \cdot min/l$$

$$(V_D)_{area} = \frac{D_0}{b \cdot [AUC]_0^\infty} = \frac{100 \, mg}{7.73 \cdot 10^{-3} \, min^{-1} \cdot 130 \, mg \cdot min/l} = 99.5 \, l$$

$$V_t = \frac{k_{12}}{k_{21}} \cdot V_P = \frac{4.32 \cdot 10^{-2}}{3.15 \cdot 10^{-2}} \cdot 35.3 \, l = 48.4 \, l$$

$$Cl_T = b \cdot (V_D)_{area} = \frac{D_0}{[AUC]_0^\infty} = \frac{100 \, mg}{130 \, mg \cdot min/l} = 0.769 \, l/min = 769 \, ml/min$$

$$Cl_T = k \cdot V_P = 2.18 \cdot 10^{-2} \, min^{-1} \cdot 35.3 \, l = 0.770 \, l/min = 770 \, ml/min$$

2.2.2 IV Infusion

In the two-compartment open model with IV drug infusion, a drug solution is infused somewhat slowly through a vein into the blood circulation and distributed rapidly throughout the central compartment, followed by a slower

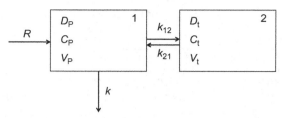

FIGURE 2.10 Two-compartment open model where the drug is administered by IV infusion and is rapidly distributed throughout the body.

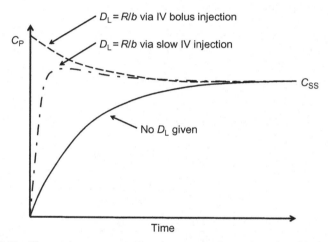

FIGURE 2.11 Plasma drug concentration–time curves for a drug that follows the two-compartment open model after IV infusion with no loading dose (D_L) or a loading dose ($D_L = R/b$) given as an IV bolus injection at $t = 0$ (*dashed line*) or as a slow IV injection (*dashed–dotted line*).

distribution into the tissue compartment (Figures 2.10 and 2.11). As before (see Section 2.1.2), the infusion rate (R) is zero order but the other rate constants are first order.

The change in the amount of drug in the body (dD_B/dt) will be:

$$\frac{dD_B}{dt} = R + k_{21} \cdot D_t - k \cdot D_B - k_{12} \cdot D_B \qquad (2.52)$$

Inserting Eqs. (2.31) and (2.32) into Eq. (2.52) and integration gives:

$$C_P = \frac{R}{V_P \cdot k} \left[1 - \left(\frac{k-b}{a-b}\right) e^{-a \cdot t} - \left(\frac{a-k}{a-b}\right) e^{-b \cdot t} \right] \qquad (2.53)$$

At steady-state (i.e., when $t = \infty$), Eq. (2.53) gives the steady-state plasma drug concentration (C_{SS}):

$$C_{SS} = \frac{R}{V_P \cdot k} \qquad (2.54)$$

Rearrangement of Eq. (2.54) gives an equation for calculating the drug infusion rate (R) for a given drug plasma concentration (C_{SS}). In the two-compartment model, the drug dose enters the central compartment (compartment 1) and is distributed rapidly throughout this compartment and then more slowly throughout the tissue compartment (compartment 2). Thus, if a loading dose (D_L) is given as an IV bolus injection, the initial plasma concentration will be much higher than C_{SS} (Figure 2.11). Even somewhat slow IV injection or multiple IV bolus injections will give drug plasma levels that are slightly higher or lower than C_{SS}.

2.3   THREE-COMPARTMENT OPEN MODEL

Three-compartment models are sometimes observed after IV bolus injections, although they are not very common. The three-compartment open model consists of three hypothetical compartments: (1) the *central compartment* (compartment 1), which represents blood, extracellular fluid, and highly perfused tissues, (2) the *tissue compartment* (compartment 2), which contains tissues in which the drug equilibrates more slowly, and (3) the *deep tissue compartment* (compartment 3), which may represent poorly perfused tissues such as bone and some fat tissue, as well as drug that is tightly bound to some specific tissues (Figure 2.12).

The three-compartment model is an extension of the two-compartment model and is described by the following equations:

$$C_P = Ae^{-a \cdot t} + Be^{-b \cdot t} + Ce^{-c \cdot t} \qquad (2.55)$$

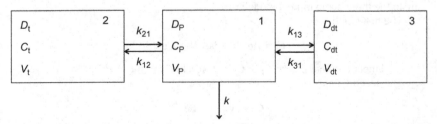

FIGURE 2.12 Three-compartment open model. The drug is administered by IV bolus injection into the central compartment (compartment 1), where it is rapidly distributed and reaches equilibrium. Then, it partitions into the tissue compartment (compartment 2), where it is more slowly equilibrated and then even more slowly into the deep tissue compartment (compartment 3).

$$[AUC]_0^\infty = \frac{A}{a} + \frac{B}{b} + \frac{C}{c} \tag{2.56}$$

$$V_P = \frac{D_0}{A + B + C} \tag{2.57}$$

$$k = \frac{a \cdot b \cdot c \cdot (A + B + C)}{A \cdot b \cdot c + B \cdot a \cdot c + C \cdot a \cdot b} \tag{2.58}$$

EXAMPLE 2.6 IV Bolus and Three-Compartment Open Model

A 70-kg man was given a single 5-mg IV bolus dose of a drug ($D_0 = 5$ mg). Blood samples were collected and the plasma concentration of the drug (C_P) determined:

Time (h)	C_p (ng/ml)
0.5	285.0
1.0	200.1
2.0	78.1
3.0	36.0
4.0	19.5
6.0	7.70
8.0	3.05
10.0	1.48
14.0	0.29
18.0	0.098
22.0	0.033
26.0	0.011

Answer

Plotting the results ($\ln C_p$ versus t) indicates that the drug is distributed according to the two- or three-compartment model. The terminal phase ($t \geq 14$ h) is linear. Then, during the next phase of calculation, a biphasic graph is observed, with a linear phase between 4 and 10 h, indicating that the drug is distributed according to the three-compartment model:

The first graph:

$$C_P = Ae^{-a \cdot t} + Be^{-b \cdot t} + Ce^{-c \cdot t}$$

Linear terminal phase: $C_P' = C \cdot e^{-c \cdot t}$ or $\ln C_P' = \ln C - c \cdot t$
The second graph:

$$C_P = Ae^{-a \cdot t} + Be^{-b \cdot t}$$

Linear terminal phase: $C_P - C_P' = C''_P = B \cdot e^{-b \cdot t}$ or $\ln C''_P = \ln B - b \cdot t$
The third graph:

$$(C_P - C_P') - C''_P = C'''_P = A \cdot e^{-a \cdot t} \text{ or } \ln C'''_P = \ln A - a \cdot t$$

Time (h)	C_P (ng/ml)	$\ln C_P$	C'_P (ng/ml)	$(C_P - C'_P)$ (ng/ml)	$\ln(C_P - C'_P)$	C''_P (ng/ml)	$(C_P - C'_P) - C''_P$ (ng/ml)	$\ln C'''_P$
0.5	285.0	5.652	11.5	273.5	5.611	98.5	175.0	5.165
1.0	200.1	5.299	10.0	190.1	5.248	75.1	115.0	4.745
2.0	78.1	4.358	7.7	70.4	4.254	43.8	26.6	3.281
3.0	36.0	3.584	5.8	30.2	3.408	25.5	4.7	1.548
4.0	19.5	2.970	4.4	15.1	2.715			
6.0	7.70	2.041	2.58	5.12	1.633			
8.0	3.05	1.115	1.49	1.56	0.445			
10.0	1.48	0.392	0.87	0.61	−0.494			
14.0	0.29	−1.238						
18.0	0.098	−2.323						
22.0	0.033	−3.411						
26.0	0.011	−4.510						

$\ln C''_P = \ln B - b \cdot t$

$\ln C'''_P = \ln A - a \cdot t$

$\ln C'_P = \ln C - c \cdot t$

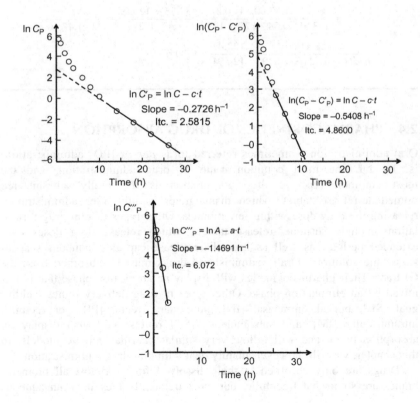

$\ln C'_P = \ln C - c \cdot t$
Slope = −0.2726 h^{-1}
Itc. = 2.5815

$\ln(C_P - C'_P) = \ln C - c \cdot t$
Slope = −0.5408 h^{-1}
Itc. = 4.8600

$\ln C'''_P = \ln A - a \cdot t$
Slope = −1.4691 h^{-1}
Itc. = 6.072

From the graph, it can be calculated that:

$A = e^{6.072} = 433.55$ ng/ml
$B = e^{4.860} = 129.02$ ng/ml
$C = e^{2.5815} = 13.22$ ng/ml
$a = 1.47$ h^{-1}
$b = 0.54$ h^{-1}
$c = 0.27$ h^{-1}

$C_P(\text{ng/ml}) = Ae^{-a \cdot t} + Be^{-b \cdot t} + Ce^{-c \cdot t} = 434 \cdot e^{-1.5 \cdot t} + 129 \cdot e^{-0.54 \cdot t} + 13.2 \cdot e^{-0.27 \cdot t}$
(t in hours)

$$[AUC]_0^\infty = \frac{A}{a} + \frac{B}{b} + \frac{C}{c} = \frac{433.55}{1.47} + \frac{129.02}{0.54} + \frac{13.22}{0.27} = 582.82 \text{ ng h/ml}$$
$$= 583 \text{ μg h/l}$$

$$V_P = \frac{D_0}{A + B + C} = \frac{5 \text{ mg}}{0.57579 \text{ mg/l}} = 8.7 \text{ l}$$

$$k = \frac{a \cdot b \cdot c \cdot (A + B + C)}{A \cdot b \cdot c + B \cdot a \cdot c + C \cdot a \cdot b}$$

$$= \frac{1.47 \cdot 0.54 \cdot 0.27 \cdot (433.55 + 129.02 + 13.22)}{433.55 \cdot 0.54 \cdot 0.27 + 129.02 \cdot 1.47 \cdot 0.27 + 13.22 \cdot 1.47 \cdot 0.54}$$

$$= \frac{123.41}{63.21 + 51.21 + 10.49} = \frac{123.41}{124.91} = 0.99 \text{ h}^{-1}$$

2.4 PHARMACOKINETICS OF DRUG ABSORPTION

Oral administration (sometimes referred to as *per os* [PO] administration) is, by far, the most common route of drug administration, and the most common type of drug formulation is the orally administered immediate-release tablet, which disintegrates rapidly after administration releasing the drug dose within few minutes. Other types of oral drug formulations include sustained-release tablets, which release drug doses over extended periods, as well as immediate-release capsules, aqueous suspensions, and solutions. Orally administered drugs must be absorbed from the GI tract. Their pharmacokinetics will display an absorption phase that is followed by an elimination phase. Other types of drug delivery routes (sublingual [SL], buccal, intranasal [IN], pulmonary, rectal [PR, per rectum], intramuscular [IM], and subcutaneous [SC] routes) will also display an absorption phase and will follow very similar pharmacokinetic models. In this chapter, we will, however, mainly deal with oral drug administration.

Drugs are only absorbed in their dissolved form. Almost all biomembranes are somewhat lipophilic, but most frequently they have an aqueous exterior. For example, mucosal surfaces are coated with a layer of aqueous mucus, ranging in thickness from less than 10 micrometers (μm) on the eye surface to about 700 μm in the intestine. Drugs must dissolve in the aqueous mucus before being absorbed through the lipophilic membranes. Thus, drug absorption depends on the physiochemical properties of the drug (e.g., its aqueous solubility, ionization, and partition coefficient from the aqueous mucus to the lipophilic epithelium) as well as on the dosage form. After it is swallowed, a tablet has to disintegrate and the solid drug particles must dissolve in the aqueous environment before the drug can be absorbed from the GI tract (Figure 2.13). Thus, drug absorption from a tablet is generally slower than from a solution or a suspension.

The drug dose in the GI tract (D_{GI}) is absorbed at a certain rate (dD_{GI}/dt) and the drug is eliminated from the body at certain rate (dD_e/dt). The difference is the rate of change of drug amount within the body (dD_B/dt).

$$\frac{dD_B}{dt} = \frac{dD_{GI}}{dt} - \frac{dD_e}{dt} \tag{2.59}$$

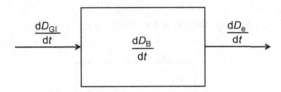

In the absorption phase, the drug is absorbed from the GI tract at a faster rate than it is eliminated from the body, and thus the amount of drug in the body (D_B) increases (Figure 2.14). In the elimination phase, the drug is eliminated from the body at a faster rate than it is absorbed, and consequently, D_B decreases. At the peak, the rate of absorption is equal to the rate of elimination. It takes some time for a tablet to disintegrate and for the solid drug particles to dissolve. Stomach emptying time and intestinal motility can also affect drug absorption. The time from administration to start of absorption is the lag time (t_L). In most cases, t_L is very short, but sometimes it can be relatively long, as, for example, in the case of enteric-coated tablets, which are designed to remain intact until they reach the intestine. Also, poorly

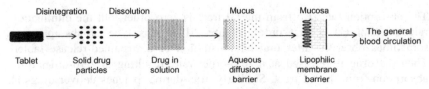

FIGURE 2.13 Drug absorption from a tablet after oral administration.

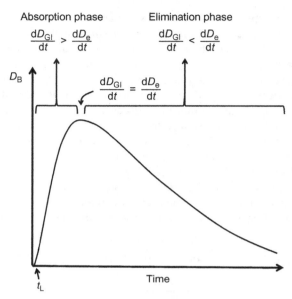

FIGURE 2.14 Drug absorption from the GI tract according to Eq. (2.59).

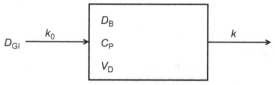

FIGURE 2.15 One-compartment open model after oral drug administration and rapid drug distributed throughout the body. k_0 is the zero-order drug absorption rate constant.

water-soluble drugs are frequently absorbed somewhat more slowly from the GI tract compared with highly water-soluble drugs, although it is harder for highly hydrophilic drugs to permeate lipophilic epithelia.

2.4.1 One-Compartment Open Model with Zero-Order Drug Absorption

The absorption rate (k_0) from the GI tract is zero order, but the elimination rate constant (k) is first order (Figure 2.15). This type of absorption is sometimes observed after oral administration of a sustained-release tablet. Then the drug is released at a zero-order rate, resulting in zero-order drug absorption from the GI tract. Similarly, transdermal patches deliver drugs at zero-order rates to the skin surface, where they are absorbed according to zero-order kinetics.

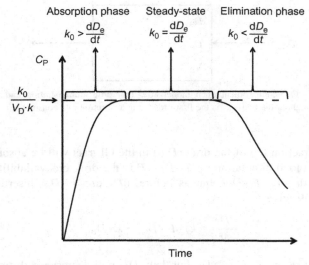

FIGURE 2.16 Drug absorption from the GI tract according to Eq. (2.62). At steady-state, $C_P = C_{SS} = k_0/V_D \cdot k$.

Here, $dD_{GI}/dt = k_0$ and $dD_e/dt = k \cdot D_B$. Inserting these into Eq. (2.59) gives:

$$\frac{dD_B}{dt} = k_0 - k \cdot D_B \tag{2.60}$$

Integration of Eq. (2.60) gives Eq. (2.61):

$$D_B = \frac{k_0}{k}(1 - e^{-k \cdot t}) \tag{2.61}$$

Or since $D_B = V_D \cdot C_P$:

$$C_P = \frac{k_0}{V_D \cdot k}(1 - e^{-k \cdot t}) \tag{2.62}$$

It is important to remember that k_0 is not the drug release rate constant (k_{rel}) from the sustained-release tablet or the transdermal patch (Figure 2.16). Only a fraction (F) of the released drug will be absorbed into the general blood circulation, and thus $k_0 = F \cdot k_{rel}$. F is the bioavailability of the drug.

2.4.2 One-Compartment Open Model with First-Order Drug Absorption

The absorption rate (k_a) from the GI tract is first order as well as the elimination rate constant (k) (Figure 2.17).

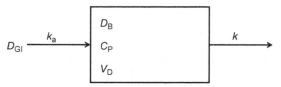

FIGURE 2.17 One-compartment open model after oral drug administration and rapid drug distributed throughout the body. k_a is the first-order drug absorption rate constant.

Only a fraction (F) of the drug (D_{GI}) in the GI tract will be absorbed into the general blood circulation, or $F \cdot D_{GI}$. F is the drug bioavailability. Thus, here, $dD_{GI}/dt = k_a \cdot F \cdot D_{GI}$, but as before, $dD_e/dt = k \cdot D_B$. Inserting these into Eq. (2.59) gives:

$$\frac{dD_B}{dt} = k_a \cdot F \cdot D_{GI} - k \cdot D_B \qquad (2.63)$$

Initially (i.e., at $t = 0$), $D_{GI} = D_0$, but then, D_{GI} will decrease with time:

$$D_{GI} = D_0 \cdot e^{-k_a \cdot t} \qquad (2.64)$$

$$\frac{dD_B}{dt} = k_a \cdot F \cdot D_0 \cdot e^{-k_a \cdot t} - k \cdot D_B \qquad (2.65)$$

Integration of Eq. (2.65) and remembering that $D_B = V_D \cdot C_P$ gives:

$$C_P = \frac{F \cdot k_a \cdot D_0}{V_D \cdot (k_a - k)} (e^{-k \cdot t} - e^{-k_a \cdot t}) \qquad (2.66)$$

C_{max} and t_{max}:

It is important to be able to calculate the maximum plasma concentration (C_{max}), sometimes called *peak plasma concentration*, and the time it takes to reach C_{max} after oral administration (t_{max}) of one dose. We know that $dD_B/dt = 0$ at t_{max} (Figure 2.14). Likewise, at t_{max} the slope of the tangent (dC_P/dt) to the C_P versus t curve is zero (Figure 2.18).

From Eq. (2.66), we get at t_{max}:

$$\frac{dC_P}{dt} = \frac{F \cdot k_a \cdot D_0}{V_D \cdot (k_a - k)} (-k \cdot e^{-k \cdot t} + k_a \cdot e^{-k_a \cdot t}) = 0 \qquad (2.67)$$

Since $(F \cdot k_a \cdot D_0)/(V_D \cdot (k_a - k)) \neq 0$ the value of $(-k \cdot e^{-k \cdot t} + k_a \cdot e^{-k_a \cdot t}) = 0$ at t_{max}. Thus, at t_{max}

$$k \cdot e^{-k \cdot t_{max}} = k_a \cdot e^{-k_a \cdot t_{max}} \qquad (2.68)$$

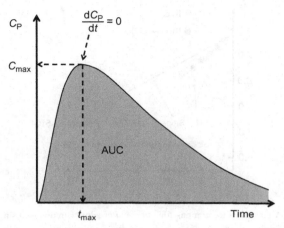

FIGURE 2.18 A plasma concentration–time curve after administration of a single oral dose. AUC is the area-under-the-curve.

Solving Eq. (2.68) for t_{max} gives Eq. (2.69):

$$t_{max} = \frac{\ln(k_a/k)}{k_a - k} \tag{2.69}$$

Then C_{max} after administration of *one* oral dose can be obtained by substituting t_{max} into Eq. (2.66).

EXAMPLE 2.7 Oral Administration and One-Compartment Open Model

A healthy male volunteer received one tablet containing 500 mg of amoxicillin. Blood samples were collected and the plasma amoxicillin concentration (C_P) determined at various time points (t). The example in based on information found in Ref. [1].

Time (h)	C_P (µg/ml)
0.50	0.01
1.00	3.23
1.50	4.44
1.75	4.28
2.0	4.20
2.5	3.64
4	3.30
5	1.18
6	0.62
7	0.31
8	0.16

Calculate k_a, k, $t_{1/2}$, t_{max}, and C_{max}.

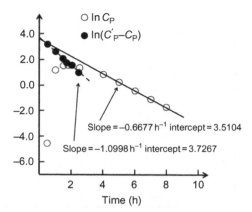

FIGURE 2.19 A plasma concentration–time curve after administration of a single oral dose of 500 mg of amoxicillin.

Answer

Plotting the ln C_P–t shows a linear elimination phase from 4 to 8 h (Figure 2.19).

Time (h)	C_P (µg/ml)	ln C_P	C_p' (µg/ml)	C_P'-C_P (µg/ml)	ln(C_P'-C_P)
0.00	0.00	—	—	—	—
0.50	0.01	−4.605	23.964	23.95	3.176
1.0	3.23	1.172	17.162	13.93	2.634
1.50	4.44	1.491	12.291	7.85	2.061
1.75	4.28	1.454	10.401	6.12	1.812
2.0	4.20	1.435	8.802	4.60	1.526
2.5	3.64	1.292	6.304	2.66	0.978
4	2.31	0.837			
5	1.18	0.166			
6	0.62	−0.478			
7	0.31	−1.171			
8	0.16	−1.833			

For rows 0.50–2.5:
$$\ln(C_P - C_P') = \ln\left(\frac{F \cdot k_a \cdot D_0}{V_D \cdot (k_a - k)}\right) - k_a \cdot t$$

For rows 4–8:
$$\ln C_P' = \ln\left(\frac{F \cdot k_a \cdot D_0}{V_D \cdot (k_a - k)}\right) - k \cdot t$$

$$\ln(C_P - C_P') = \ln\left(\frac{F \cdot k_a \cdot D_0}{V_D \cdot (k_a - k)}\right) - k_a \cdot t$$

The values of the rate constants are obtained from the slopes:

Slope $= -k_a = -1.0998\ \text{h}^{-1}$ or $k_a = 1.10\ \text{h}^{-1}$

Slope $= -k = -0.6677\ \text{h}^{-1}$ or $k = 0.67\ \text{h}^{-1}$

Then, technically, the Y-intercepts of the two lines should be identical and equal to $\ln((F \cdot k_a \cdot D_0)/(V_D \cdot (k_a - k)))$, but they are not, partly due to the lag time and partly due to the method applied (called *residuals* or *feathering technique*) to obtain the rate constants. The line of the elimination phase is based on the origi-nal experimental values, and its slope is smaller than the line of the absorption phase, which is based on the residual concentrations; that is, the values are obtained by subtracting the experimental values from the values of the extrapo-lated values of the elimination phase ($C'_P - C_P$). Consequently, the elimination phase Y-intercept is frequently more accurate and thus used to calculate the intercept.

$$\ln C'_P = \ln\left(\frac{F \cdot k_a \cdot D_0}{V_D \cdot (k_a - k)}\right) - k \cdot t = \ln B - k \cdot t = 3.51 - 0.67 \cdot t$$

$$\ln(C_P - C'_P) = \ln\left(\frac{F \cdot k_a \cdot D_0}{V_D \cdot (k_a - k)}\right) - k_a \cdot t = \ln A - k_a \cdot t = 3.73 - 1.10 \cdot t$$

The equation describes the plasma concentration–time curve after adminis-tration, and the 500 mg amoxicillin tablet will then be:

$$C_P = \frac{F \cdot k_a \cdot D_0}{V_D \cdot (k_a - k)}(e^{-k \cdot t} - e^{-k_a \cdot t}) = e^{3.51} \cdot (e^{-0.67 \cdot t} - e^{-1.10 \cdot t})$$
$$= 33.4 \cdot (e^{-0.67 \cdot t} - e^{-1.10 \cdot t})$$

Alternatively, the equation can be written as follows:

$$C_P = Be^{-k \cdot t} - Ae^{-k_a \cdot t} \tag{2.70}$$

$$C_P = e^{3.51} \cdot e^{-0.67 \cdot t} - e^{3.73} \cdot e^{-1.10 \cdot t} = 33.4 \cdot e^{-0.67 \cdot t} - 41.7 \cdot e^{-1.10 \cdot t}$$

The half-life is generally calculated as follows:

$$t_{1/2} = \frac{\ln 2}{k} = \frac{0.693}{0.67 \text{ h}^{-1}} = 1.0 \text{ h}$$

However, in the elimination phase, the rate of drug absorption is slower than the rate of drug elimination (Eq. (2.59) and Figure 2.14). Although C_P is decreasing during the elimination phase, some drug is still being absorbed from the GI tract, especially at the beginning of the phase, making $t_{1/2}$ obtained somewhat inaccurate. Thus, reported $t_{1/2}$ values are generally based on data col-lected after IV bolus injections, where drug absorption does not interfere with determination of the drug elimination constants. Value of t_{max} is calculated from Eq. (2.69):

$$t_{max} = \frac{\ln(k_a/k)}{k_a - k} = \frac{\ln(1.10/0.67)}{1.10 - 0.67} = 1.2 \text{ h}$$

We can then use this t_{max} to calculate C_{max}, according to either Eq. (2.66) or Eq. (2.70):

$$C_{max} = \frac{F \cdot k_a \cdot D_0}{V_D \cdot (k_a - k)}(e^{-k \cdot t_{max}} - e^{-k_a \cdot t_{max}}) = e^{3.51} \cdot (e^{-0.67 \cdot 1.2} - e^{-1.10 \cdot 1.2}) = 6.0 \text{ μg/ml}$$

or

$$C_{max} = 33.4 \cdot e^{-0.67 \cdot t_{max}} - 41.7 \cdot e^{-1.10 \cdot t_{max}} = 33.4 \cdot 0.4475 - 41.7 \cdot 0.2671$$
$$= 3.8 \text{ μg/ml}$$

The observed t_{max} and C_{max} values in the data table of Example 2.7 are 1.5 h and 4.4 μg/ml, respectively. Equation (2.70) accounts for lag time and gives C_{max} value that is closer to the observed value.

2.4.3 One-Compartment Open Model with Urine Sample Collection

As before, the absorption rate (k_a) from the GI tract is first order as well as the elimination rate constant (k) (Figure 2.17), but k is the sum of the first-order rate constant for urinary excretion of the unmetabolized drug (k_e) and the first-order nonrenal rate constant (k_{nr}):

$$k = k_e + k_{nr} \tag{2.71}$$

k_{nr} is composed of other rate constants such as the first-order metabolic rate constant (k_m) and the first-order rate constant for biliary excretion (k_b). From Eq. (2.66) we get:

$$D_B = \frac{F \cdot k_a \cdot D_0}{(k_a - k)} (e^{-k \cdot t} - e^{-k_a \cdot t}) \tag{2.72}$$

Combining Eqs. (2.17) and (2.72) gives:

$$\frac{dD_U}{dt} = \frac{F \cdot k_e \cdot k_a \cdot D_0}{(k_a - k)} (e^{-k \cdot t} - e^{-k_a \cdot t}) \tag{2.73}$$

Plotting $\ln(\Delta D_U / \Delta t)$ versus t gives the curve shown in Figure 2.20, where ΔD_U is the amount of drug excreted with urine during a given period (Δt) and t is the time at middle of the collection period. The feathering technique can be applied to calculate k_a and k:

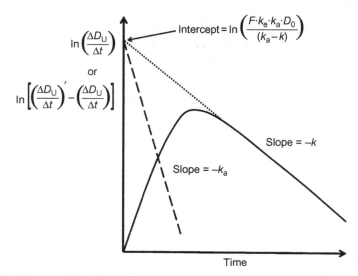

FIGURE 2.20 A $\ln(\Delta D_U / \Delta t)$ versus t plot gives the curve and then the rate constants are obtained, as shown in Example 2.7.

$$\ln\left(\frac{\Delta D_U}{\Delta t}\right)' = \ln\left(\frac{F \cdot k_e \cdot k_a \cdot D_0}{(k_a - k)}\right) - k \cdot t \tag{2.74}$$

$$\ln\left[\left(\frac{\Delta D_U}{\Delta t}\right)' - \left(\frac{\Delta D_U}{\Delta t}\right)\right] = \ln\left(\frac{F \cdot k_e \cdot k_a \cdot D_0}{k_a - k}\right) - k_a \cdot t \tag{2.75}$$

Alternatively, Eq. (2.72) can be integrated:

$$\int_0^{D_U} dD_U = \frac{F \cdot k_e \cdot k_a \cdot D_0}{(k_a - k)} \int_0^t (e^{-k \cdot t} - e^{-k_a \cdot t}) dt \tag{2.76}$$

Giving us Eq. (2.77):

$$D_U = \frac{F \cdot k_e \cdot k_a \cdot D_0}{(k_a - k)}\left(\frac{e^{-k_a \cdot t}}{k_a} - \frac{e^{-k \cdot t}}{k}\right) + \frac{F \cdot k_e \cdot D_0}{k} \tag{2.77}$$

$$\text{urine} = D_U^\infty = \frac{F \cdot k_e \cdot D_0}{k} \tag{2.78}$$

EXAMPLE 2.8 Oral Administration and Urine Sample Collection

A healthy male volunteer received one tablet containing 500 mg of amoxicillin (see Example 2.7). The bioavailability (F) of amoxicillin after oral administration was determined to be 90%. Urine samples were collected and the cumulative amount of amoxicillin in urine determined (Figure 2.21). Determine k_e. The example in based on information found in Ref. [1].

From Figure 2.21, we can estimate that $D_U^\infty = F \cdot k_e \cdot D_0/k = 260$ mg or

$$k_e = \frac{D_U^\infty \cdot k}{F \cdot D_0} = \frac{260 \text{ mg} \cdot 0.67 \text{ h}^{-1}}{0.90 \cdot 500 \text{ mg}} = 0.39 \text{ h}^{-1}$$

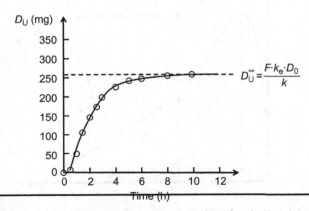

FIGURE 2.21 Cumulative urinary drug excretion versus time after single oral dose.

2.4.4 Two-Compartment Open Model with First-Order Drug Absorption

When a drug follows a two-compartment open model with first-order absorption, after oral administration, the drug dose is absorbed from the GI tract into the blood circulation and distributed very rapidly throughout the central compartment and then more slowly throughout the tissue compartment (Figures 2.22 and 2.23). The GI tract, as well as the kidneys, liver, and other highly perfused tissues such as the heart, lungs, and brain, belongs to the central compartment. Thus, the drug both enters and leaves the body via the central compartment. The tissue compartment comprises less perfused tissues such as muscle, fat, and skin. The equation for C_P versus time profile for a drug that follows the two-compartment model with first-order drug absorption is obtained by adding an absorption phase to Eq. (2.35):

$$C_P = Ae^{-a \cdot t} + Be^{-b \cdot t} - Ce^{-k_a \cdot t} \tag{2.79}$$

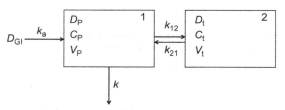

FIGURE 2.22 Two-compartment open model after oral drug administration. The drug is absorbed into the central compartment (compartment 1), where it is rapidly distributed and reaches equilibrium. Then, it partitions into the tissue compartment (compartment), where it is more slowly equilibrated. k_a is the first-order drug absorption rate constant.

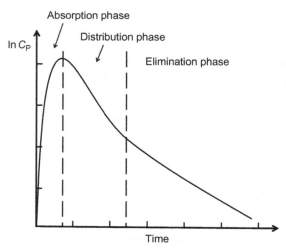

FIGURE 2.23 The ln C_P—time profile after oral drug administration. The drug pharmacokinetics follows the two-compartment open model.

The values of the constants A, B, C, a, b, and k_a are obtained by using the feathering technique (see Example 2.9).

EXAMPLE 2.9 Oral Administration and Two-Compartment Model

A drug dose of 20 mg was given to a healthy volunteer, blood samples collected, and the drug plasma concentration determined. Calculate A, B, C, a, b, and k_a.

Time (h)	C_P (ng/ml)	Time (h)	C_P (ng/ml)	Time (h)	C_P (ng/ml)
0.5	21.2	15	37.5	40	11.5
1.0	35.9	20	27.4	50	8.1
5.0	68.5	25	20.9	60	6.0
10	52.4	30	17.1		

Answer

As in Examples 2.6 and 2.7, we apply the feathering technique:

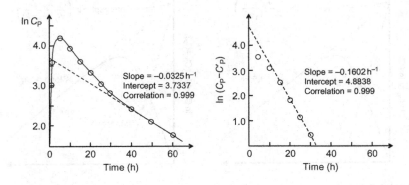

	Time (h)	C_P (ng/ml)	ln C_P	$(C_P - C_P')$ (ng/ml)	$\ln(C_P - C_P')$	$C_P'' - (C_P - C_P')$ (ng/ml)	$\ln(C_P'' - (C_P - C_P'))$
Absorption	0.5	21.2	3.054	−20.0	−	142.0	4.956
	1.0	35.9	3.581	−4.6	−	117.2	4.764
	5.0	68.5	4.227	32.9	3.493	26.4	3.273
	10	52.4	3.959	22.2	3.100	4.4	1.482
Distrubution	15	37.5	3.624	11.8	2.468		
	20	27.4	3.311	5.6	1.723		
	25	20.9	3.040	2.3	0.833		
	30	17.1	2.839	1.1	0.095		
Elimination	40	11.5	2.442				
	50	8.1	2.092				
	60	6.0	1.792				

$$C_P'' - (C_P - C_P') = C \cdot e^{-k_a \cdot t} \text{ or}$$
$$\ln(C_P'' - (C_P - C_P')) = \ln C - k_a \cdot t$$

$$C_P' = B \cdot e^{-b \cdot t} \text{ or}$$
$$\ln C_P' = \ln B - b \cdot t$$

$$C_P'' = (C_P - C_P') = A \cdot e^{-a \cdot t} \text{ or}$$
$$\ln C_P'' = \ln(C_P - C_P') = \ln A - a \cdot t$$

Slope = −0.0325 h⁻¹
Intercept = 3.7337
Correlation = 0.999

Slope = −0.1602 h⁻¹
Intercept = 4.8838
Correlation = 0.999

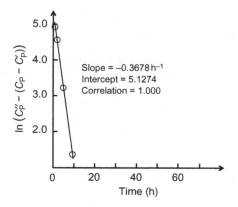

$A = e^{4.8838} = 132.1$ ng/ml; $B = e^{3.7337} = 41.8$ ng/ml; $C = e^{5.1274} = 168.6$ ng/ml;
$a = 0.16$ h^{-1}; $b = 3.3 \times 10^{-2}$ h^{-1}; $k_a = 0.37$ h^{-1}

or

$C_P = Ae^{-a \cdot t} + Be^{-b \cdot t} - Ce^{-k_a \cdot t} = 132.1e^{-0.16 \cdot t} + 41.8e^{-0.033 \cdot t} - 168.6e^{-0.37 \cdot t}$
(ng/ml), where t is in hours.

2.4.5 Flip-Flop Pharmacokinetics

Flip-flop pharmacokinetics can be observed when drug is absorbed more slowly into the general blood circulation than it is eliminated from the circulation (i.e., when $k > k_a$). This can be the case if, for example, the drug has unusually short biologic half-life ($t_{1/2} < 1$ h) or when a drug is given as an extended-release product (Figure 2.24). Comparing the k-value obtained

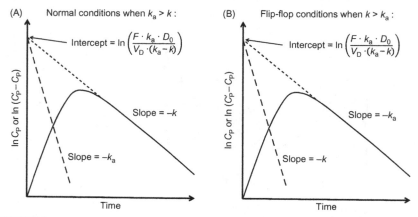

FIGURE 2.24   Flip-flop when feathering technique (the method of residuals) is used to determine k and k_a.

from an oral product with one obtained after IV bolus injection of the drug can give some idea whether flip-flop pharmacokinetics has occurred. Alternatively, k_a can be determined by plotting the percentage of drug unabsorbed versus time (the Wagner-Nelson method) [2].

2.5 BIOAVAILABILITY

Most commonly, the term *bioavailability* is used to describe the fraction of administered drug dose that reaches the systemic blood circulation in its intact (i.e., unmetabolized) form after, for example, oral administration. By definition, the bioavailability of intravenously administered drug is 100%. After extravascular administration (e.g., after oral, nasal, buccal, or dermal administration), drug bioavailability is most often less than 100% due to, for example, incomplete absorption or first-pass metabolism. *Absolute availability (F)* of a drug is its systemic availability after extravascular administration compared with IV dosing of the same drug. F is the fraction of drug absorbed from, for example, the GI tract after oral administration and is based on the dose-corrected AUC that is obtained from plasma drug concentration versus time (C_P versus t) plots:

$$F = \frac{[\text{AUC}]_{\text{PO}}/\text{Dose}_{\text{PO}}}{[\text{AUC}]_{\text{IV}}/\text{Dose}_{\text{IV}}} \tag{2.80}$$

AUC from time zero to infinity ($t = 0 - \infty$) is:

$$[\text{AUC}]_0^\infty = \int_0^\infty C_P \, dt \tag{2.81}$$

For the one-compartment model and IV bolus injection, Eq. (2.5) is inserted into Eq. (2.81):

$$[\text{AUC}]_0^\infty = \frac{D_0}{V_D} \int_0^\infty e^{-k \cdot t} dt = \frac{D_0}{V_D \cdot k} \tag{2.82}$$

For the one-compartment model and oral administration with first-order absorption, Eq. (2.66) is inserted into Eq. (2.81):

$$[\text{AUC}]_0^\infty = \frac{F \cdot k_a \cdot D_0}{V_D \cdot (k_a - k)} \int_0^\infty (e^{-k \cdot t} - e^{-k_a \cdot t}) dt = \frac{F \cdot k_a \cdot D_0}{V_D \cdot (k_a - k)} \left(\frac{1}{k} - \frac{1}{k_a} \right)$$

$$= \frac{F \cdot D_0}{V_D \cdot k} \tag{2.83}$$

Alternatively, Eq. (2.70) can be inserted into Eq. (2.81) to obtain:

$$[\text{AUC}]_0^\infty = \int_0^\infty (Be^{-k \cdot t} - Ae^{-k_a \cdot t}) dt = \frac{B}{k} - \frac{A}{k_a} \tag{2.84}$$

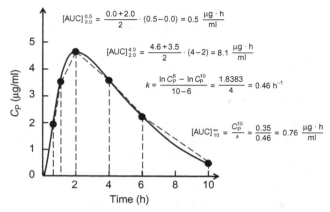

FIGURE 2.25 Estimation of the AUC after oral drug administration by the trapezoidal method. $[\text{AUC}]_0^\infty = 0.50 + 1.38 + 4.05 + 8.10 + 5.70 + 7.48 + 0.76 = 28.0 \ \mu\text{g} \cdot \text{h/ml}$.

For the two-compartment model and oral administration with first-order absorption, Eq. (2.79) is inserted into Eq. (2.81):

$$[\text{AUC}]_0^\infty = \int_0^\infty (Ae^{-a \cdot t} + Be^{-b \cdot t} - Ce^{-k_a \cdot t}) \mathrm{d}t = \frac{A}{a} + \frac{B}{b} - \frac{C}{k_a} \qquad (2.85)$$

Equation (2.51) is used to calculate AUC for a drug following the two-compartment model after IV bolus injection, and Eq. (2.56) is used to calculate the AUC for a drug following the three-compartment model after IV bolus injection. The AUC can also be calculated by a model-independent method called *trapezoidal method*, in which the AUC is estimated by dividing the C_P versus t curve into several trapezoids (Figure 2.25).

Relative availability (F_{rel}) is the drug availability from a product compared with that from another product given by the same route, for example, by comparing the AUC for a tablet (A) and the AUC for the same drug in solution (B) after oral administration:

$$F_{\text{rel}} = \frac{[\text{AUC}]_A / \text{Dose}_A}{[\text{AUC}]_B / \text{Dose}_B} \qquad (2.86)$$

EXAMPLE 2.10 Absolute Availability of Midazolam Nasal Spray

The absolute availability of nasally administered midazolam (in a parenteral solution) was determined in eight healthy individuals. The IV bolus dose (D_{IV}) was 2 mg and the intranasal dose (D_{IN}) was 19.5 mg. Blood samples were taken at various time intervals and the plasma concentration of the drug (C_P) determined [3]. Calculate the absolute availability of midazolam in a nasal spray.

Time (min)	C_P (ng/ml)	
	IV bolus	IN
5	118	89.2
10	88.0	121
20	70.4	136
30	39.3	123
45	27.8	110
60	20.4	98.0
90	14.5	78.5
120	12.1	65.3
180	9.58	47.2
240	7.58	34.0
360	4.93	23.1

Answer

Midazolam is distributed according to the two-compartment open model after IV and nasal administration, and the data in the table above were used to obtain the following equations:

$$\text{IV: } C_P = A \cdot e^{-a \cdot t} + B \cdot e^{-b \cdot t} = 127 \cdot e^{-5.23 \cdot 10^{-2} \text{min}^{-1} \cdot t} + 18.7 \cdot e^{-3.73 \cdot 10^{-3} \text{min}^{-1} \cdot t} \text{ ng/ml}$$

$$\text{IN: } C_P = A \cdot e^{-a \cdot t} + B \cdot e^{-b \cdot t} - C \cdot e^{-k_a \cdot t} = 90.5 \cdot e^{-1.5 \cdot 10^{-2} \text{min}^{-1} \cdot t} + 73.6 \cdot e^{-3.22 \cdot 10^{-3} \text{min}^{-1} \cdot t}$$
$$- 161.6 \cdot e^{-0.176 \text{ min}^{-1} \cdot t} \text{ ng/ml}$$

AUC from time zero to infinity is then calculated according to Eqs. (2.51) and (2.85):

$$\text{IV: } [AUC]_0^\infty = \frac{A}{a} + \frac{B}{b} = \frac{127 \text{ ng/ml}}{5.23 \cdot 10^{-2} \text{ min}^{-1}} + \frac{18.7 \text{ ng/ml}}{3.73 \cdot 10^{-3} \text{ min}^{-1}}$$
$$= 7471 \text{ ng} \cdot \text{min/ml}$$

$$\text{IN: } [AUC]_0^\infty = \frac{A}{a} + \frac{B}{b} - \frac{C}{k_a} = \frac{90.5 \text{ ng/ml}}{1.50 \cdot 10^{-2} \text{ min}^{-1}} + \frac{73.6 \text{ ng/ml}}{3.22 \cdot 10^{-3} \text{ min}^{-1}}$$
$$- \frac{161.6 (\text{ng/ml})}{0.176 \text{ min}^{-1}} = 27,972 \text{ ng} \cdot \text{min/ml}$$

Absolute availability is then calculated according to Eq. (2.80):

$$F = \frac{[AUC]_{IN}/Dose_{IN}}{[AUC]_{IV}/Dose_{IV}} = \frac{27,972/19.5}{7,471/2} = 0.39 \text{ or } 39\%$$

EXAMPLE 2.11 Relative Availability

The relative availability of a drug in a tablet was determined in 18 healthy individuals with a solution of the same drug as a reference formulation. The drug dose was 500 mg in both cases. Blood samples were taken at various time intervals and the plasma concentration of the drug (C_P) determined. Calculate the relative availability of the drug in the tablets.

Time (min)	C_P (μg/ml)	
	Oral solution	Oral tablets
20	4.49	1.44
40	5.43	2.05
60	5.14	2.33
120	3.16	2.22
180	1.63	1.71
240	0.79	1.15
300	0.40	0.78
360	0.19	0.48
720	0.01	0.02

Answer

The drug is distributed according to the one-compartment open model with first-order drug absorption after oral administration. The C_P versus time profile is shown in the figure below. The experimental data was fitted to Eq. (2.66) and the AUC calculated according to Eq. (2.83).

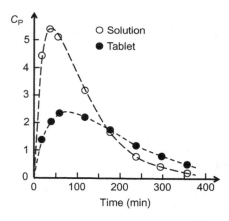

Solution:

$$C_P = \frac{F \cdot k_a \cdot D_0}{V_D \cdot (k_a - k)}(e^{-k \cdot t} - e^{-k_a \cdot t}) = 12.90 \ \mu g/ml \cdot (e^{-1.16 \cdot 10^{-2} \cdot t} - e^{-3.71 \cdot 10^{-2} \cdot t})$$

$$[AUC]_0^\infty = \frac{F \cdot k_a \cdot D_0}{V_D \cdot (k_a - k)}\left(\frac{1}{k} - \frac{1}{k_a}\right) = 12.90 \cdot \left(\frac{1}{1.16 \cdot 10^{-2}} - \frac{1}{3.71 \cdot 10^{-2}}\right)$$
$$= 7.64 \cdot 10^2 \ \mu g \ min \ ml^{-1}$$

Tablet:

$$C_P = \frac{F \cdot k_a \cdot D_0}{V_D \cdot (k_a - k)}(e^{-k \cdot t} - e^{-k_a \cdot t}) = 8.77 \ \mu g/ml \cdot (e^{-8.37 \cdot 10^{-3} \cdot t} - e^{-1.74 \cdot 10^{-2} \cdot t})$$

$$[AUC]_0^\infty = \frac{F \cdot k_a \cdot D_0}{V_D \cdot (k_a - k)}\left(\frac{1}{k} - \frac{1}{k_a}\right) = 8.77 \cdot \left(\frac{1}{8.37 \cdot 10^{-3}} - \frac{1}{1.74 \cdot 10^{-2}}\right)$$
$$= 5.44 \cdot 10^2 \ \mu g \ min \ ml^{-1}$$

The two k-values (i.e., $1.16 \cdot 10^{-2}$ and $8.37 \cdot 10^{-3}$ min^{-1}) should, in theory, be identical, but they are not. It is important to remember that the drug is still absorbed in the elimination phase (see Section 2.4), and since the drug is absorbed about two times slower from the tablet than from the solution ($3.71 \cdot 10^{-2}/1.74 \cdot 10^{-2} \approx 2$) the observed elimination rate constant (k) for the tablet is significantly smaller than the observed elimination rate constant for the solution. Finally, Eq. (2.86) is applied to calculate the relative availability:

$$F_{rel} = \frac{[AUC]_{Tablet}/Dose_{Tablet}}{[AUC]_{Solution}/Dose_{Solution}} = \frac{544/500}{764/500} = 0.712 \text{ or } 71.2\%$$

Since, by definition, the drug in aqueous solution has 100% pharmaceutical availability when given orally, the *pharmaceutical availability* of the tablet is only 71.2%. By appropriate formulation, it should be possible to increase the drug availability from the tablet.

It can be calculated (Eq. (2.69)) that t_{max} for the solution is 46 min, whereas it is 81 min for the tablet, and C_{max} (Eq. (2.66)) is 5.22 μg/ml for the solution and 2.31 μg/ml for the tablet.

In general, two oral drug products containing the same drug are said to be *bioequivalent* only if they have close to identical AUC, t_{max}, and C_{max}. Two products with identical AUCs have the same bioavailability, but to be bioequivalent, the C_P versus t profiles have to be close to identical. Only then can the two products be expected to be, for all practical purposes, identical. If the AUCs for two products are identical but the t_{max} and C_{max} values are different, the products will have identical bioavailability, although the products are not bioequivalent (Figure 2.26).

Bioavailability can be calculated from urinary excretion data, either from the rate of drug excretion (Figure 2.27B), that is, from the AUC calculated from Eqs. (2.18) and (2.73), or from the cumulative amount of drug excreted in urine (Figure 2.27C), according to Eqs. (2.87) and (2.88):

$$F = \frac{D_{PO}^\infty/Dose_{PO}}{D_{IV}^\infty/Dose_{IV}} \qquad (2.87)$$

$$F_{rel} = \frac{D_A^\infty/Dose_A}{D_B^\infty/Dose_B} \qquad (2.88)$$

From Figure 2.27C, it can be seen that the oral solution has $F \approx 0.80$, whereas the tablet has $F \approx 0.55$. If the solution is the reference formulation, then the tablet has $F_{rel} \approx 0.55/0.80 \approx 0.7$. Since the solution has 100% pharmaceutical availability, by definition, but only 80% absolute availability, the biologic availability of the drug is 80%, which will be the maximum oral

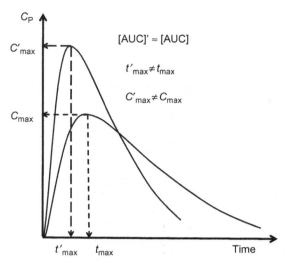

FIGURE 2.26 C_P versus t profiles of a drug in two different drug products (e.g., tablet and capsule). The products have identical bioavailability, that is $F_{rel} \approx 1.0$, but since both their t_{max} and C_{max} are different, they cannot be considered bioequivalent.

bioavailability of the drug (Figure 1.1). In other words, through appropriate reformulation of the tablet, the absolute availability can possibly be increased from 55% to the maximum of 80%. To exceed 80% bioavailability, the physicochemical properties of the drug itself have to be changed (e.g., through prodrug formation), or the drug absorption barrier within the body has to be temporary decreased (e.g., by co-administration of enzyme inhibitors).

Bioavailability studies are conducted to determine the pharmacokinetic parameters of new chemical entities and to determine the linearity of bioavailability parameters over proposed clinical dose range, inter- and intrasubject variability, and effect of food and co-administered drugs; bioequivalence studies, however, are conducted to test the effect of the formulation and its excipients on drug availability during formulation development and marketing of a generic drug product. Typically, 12 or more healthy subjects participate in bioavailability and bioequivalence studies. Generally, a crossover design is used, and each subject receives different products during different periods. In that case, the subjects cross over from one drug product to another during the course of the study, with sufficient time allowed between study periods to allow drug elimination from the body of the study subject (Table 2.2). In a Latin-square crossover design, each subject receives each product only once and serves as his or her own control, thus minimizing intersubject variation as well as variations due to, for example, product sequencing.

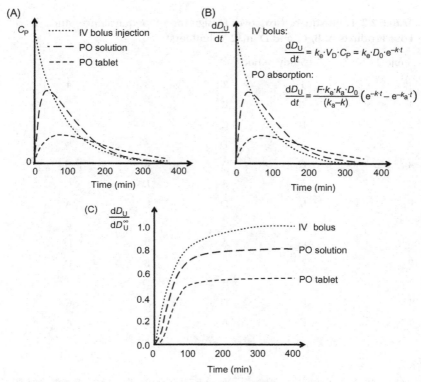

FIGURE 2.27 Sketches of a plasma concentration versus time profile (**A**) and the corresponding rate of drug urinary excretion versus time profile (**B**) and a corresponding sketch of the cumulative amount of drug excreted in urine (**C**). Note that since the urinary excretion rate is proportional to C_P, the profiles in Figures A and B have identical shapes, although the units of the Y-axis are different.

2.6   DRUG DISTRIBUTION, PROTEIN BINDING, AND CLEARANCE

After drug absorption into the general blood circulation, the drug molecules are distributed throughout the body, and eventually reach their site of action. Drug distribution within the body is, for example, dependent on the regional blood flow, the ability of the drug molecules to permeate biologic membranes such as the blood vessel walls, the drug's lipophilicity, and the drug binding to tissue and plasma proteins. In general, drugs are readily distributed to highly perfused organs such as the kidneys, heart, and liver, but are distributed more slowly to less perfused organs such as muscles and fat (Table 2.3). Drug distribution becomes *flow limited* if the drug molecules permeate readily biologic membranes but *permeability limited* if the molecules permeate membranes slowly. Since the kidneys are highly perfused

TABLE 2.2 Latin-square Crossover Design for a Bioequivalence Study of Four Products A, B, C, and D in 12 Volunteers

Subject	Study period			
	1	2	3	4
1	A	B	C	D
2	B	C	D	A
3	C	D	A	B
4	D	A	B	C
5	A	B	D	C
6	B	D	C	A
7	D	C	A	B
8	C	A	B	D
9	A	C	B	D
10	C	B	D	A
11	B	D	A	C
12	D	A	C	B

TABLE 2.3 Approximate Cardiac Output and Blood Flow

Tissue	Cardiac output (%)	Blood flow (ml/min per 100 g tissue)
Kidneys	24	450
Heart	4	70
Brain	13	55
Liver	10	25
Skin	5	5
Skeletal muscle	15	3
Fat	2	1

organs, and since most low-molecular-weight drugs readily permeate the glomerular filtration membrane, decreased cardiac output (i.e., volume of blood being pumped by the heart per unit time) will decrease the renal clearance of a drug through reduced blood flow and filtration pressure. Likewise decreased cardiac output can decrease drug uptake by the liver. In contrast, inflammation and diseases that augment capillary membrane permeability can increase the distribution volume of drugs that are permeability limited.

2.6.1 Protein Binding

After the drug molecules have been absorbed into plasma or after they have been injected into the blood circulation, the drug molecules are carried by the blood circulation to the target tissue within the body where they bind to receptors (Figure 2.28). The drug molecules are also carried to the eliminating organs such as the liver and kidneys. Plasma proteins and the various body tissues are able to bind drug molecules through the formation of drug—protein complexes. Formation of such complexes is reversible and is normally referred to as *drug—protein binding*. Drug—protein binding does affect the ability of drug molecules to permeate biologic membranes and their ability to interact with enzymes and receptors. Only unbound drug molecules permeate membrane barriers and interact with drug receptors or undergo metabolism and glomerular filtration, and thus drug—protein binding will affect the drug's pharmacokinetics (Figure 2.28). In general, decreased concentration of free drug due to protein binding will decrease the glomerular filtration rate (GFR) as well as enzymatic drug degradation, both of which will result in increased $t_{1/2}$. The most common type of plasma protein binding is formation of a drug complex with human serum albumin

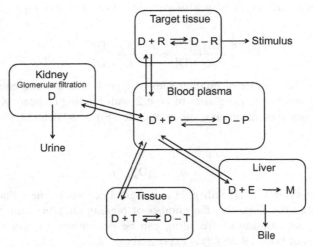

FIGURE 2.28 Drug distribution from plasma to various tissues. Only the unbound drug (D) molecules are able to permeate the biomembranes. Drug bound to plasma proteins (P) or tissue (T) is unable to permeate the membranes. Also, only the unbound drug molecules are able to bind to enzymes (E) and to receptors (R) to produce stimulus leading to pharmacologic response.

(HSA) [4,5]. HSA consists of 585 amino acid residues and has a molecular weight of 66.5 kilodaltons (kDa). Normal plasma concentration of HSA is between 35 and 55 mg/ml, but it varies with age, exercise, stress, and disease. It is a nonspecific complexing agent that acts as a solubilizer of poorly water-soluble drugs. HSA and other plasma proteins may possess several binding sites (i.e., each protein molecule may bind several drug molecules):

$$D + P \rightleftarrows D - P \text{ and } D + D - P \rightleftarrows D_2 - P \text{ and } D + D_2 - P \rightleftarrows D_3 - P \text{ and so on.}$$

If only one binding site exists, then:

$$P + D \overset{K}{\rightleftarrows} PD \tag{2.89}$$

$$r = \frac{\text{concentration of bound drug}}{\text{total concentration of protein}} = \frac{[D - P]}{[D - P] + [P]} = \frac{[D - P]}{[P]_T} = \frac{K \cdot [D]}{1 + K \cdot [D]} \tag{2.90}$$

where K is the binding constant or the equilibrium constant of the complex formation, $[P]$ is the concentration of free protein, $[D-P]$ is the concentration of the drug−protein complex, and $[D]$ is the concentration of free drug. However, since each protein has n number of independent binding sites, we get:

$$r = \frac{\text{concentration of bound drug}}{\text{total concentration of protein}} = \frac{n \cdot K \cdot [D]}{1 + K \cdot [D]} \tag{2.91}$$

Large protein molecules may also contain more than one type of binding sites:

$$r = \frac{n_1 \cdot K_1 \cdot [D]}{1 + K_1 \cdot [D]} + \frac{n_2 \cdot K_2 \cdot [D]}{1 + K_2 \cdot [D]} + \cdots \tag{2.92}$$

where n_1 is the number of binding sites of type 1 with binding constant K_1, n_2 is the number of binding sites of type 2 with binding constant K_2, and so on. If only one type of binding site exists, then Eq. (2.91) can be rewritten to give:

$$\frac{1}{r} = \frac{1}{n \cdot K} \cdot \frac{1}{[D]} + \frac{1}{n} \tag{2.93}$$

Plotting $1/r$ against $1/[D]$ will give a straight line, where the value of K is obtained from the slope and the number of binding sites (n) from the intercept. The concentration of free drug can be determined by using dialysis. The fraction of bound drug (β) is expressed as:

$$\beta = \frac{\text{concentration of bound drug}}{\text{total concentration of drug}} = \frac{[PD]}{[PD] + [D]} = \frac{n \cdot K \cdot [P]_T}{1 + K \cdot [D] + n \cdot K \cdot [P]_T} \tag{2.94}$$

The plasma protein binding is nonlinear, and thus the fraction of bound drug is dependent on the concentration of both the drug and the protein. Drugs with high K-value may saturate the protein, resulting in a decrease in β-values with increasing drug concentration. Drugs with relatively high β-values are susceptible to drug–drug interactions due to competitive drug–protein binding. In general, lipophilic drugs display higher β-value compared with hydrophilic drugs, and V_D decreases with increasing β-values (only unbound drug is able to permeate capillary walls). Since only free drug is excreted in urine by glomerular filtration, the fraction of drug excreted with urine decreases with increasing β-values. Furthermore, protein binding decreases enzymatic degradation of drugs. Thus, $t_{1/2}$ tends to increase with increasing β-values. These relationships between protein binding and other pharmacokinetic parameters are usually best observed for closely related analogs such as tetracyclines (Table 2.4). The lipophilicity of a drug will also affect its tissue distribution. For example, the more lipophilic tetracyclines (e.g., minocycline and doxycycline) partition more effectively into the sebaceous follicles compared with the more hydrophilic ones and thus are favored in the treatment of acne.

2.6.2 Clearance

Drugs are cleared (i.e., excreted) from the body through various routes of elimination, mainly as intact drug molecules, or through metabolism. The

TABLE 2.4 Lipophilicity (log $P_{octanol/water}$), Plasma Protein Binding (β), Elimination Half-Life ($t_{1/2}$), Apparent Volume of Distribution (V_D) as Liters Per kg Body Weight, and Fraction Eliminated with Urine (f_e) of Some Tetracycline Analogs in Humans

Tetracycline analog	Log $P_{O/W}$[a]	β[b]	$t_{1/2}$ (h)	V_D (l/kg)	f_e[c]
Oxytetracycline	−1.6	0.20−0.35	9	1.4	0.7
Tetracycline	−1.3	0.25−0.65	6−12	1.3	0.6
Demeclocycline	−1.3	0.40−0.50	10−15	1.7	0.4
Chlortetracycline	−0.9	0.50−0.55	6	1.6	0.2
Minocycline	0.05	0.70−0.75	11−22	1.3	0.1
Methacycline	−0.4	0.80−0.95	14−15	0.95	0.3
Doxycycline	−0.02	0.82−0.90	22	0.75	0.4

[a]Logarithm of the partition coefficient between octanol and water (pH ≈ 7.4).
[b]Fraction of drug that is protein bound in plasma.
[c]Fraction of drug excreted unchanged with urine.
The data were collected from Refs. [6−9].

intact drug is mainly excreted in urine (renal clearance, Cl_R) but is also eliminated in the bile fluid (biliary clearance, Cl_B) as well as in other body fluids such as sweat, saliva, and milk (in lactating women). In addition intact volatile compounds (e.g., gaseous anesthetics) are excreted from the lungs in expired air. Drug metabolism is sometimes referred to as *biotransformation* and occurs mainly in the liver (hepatic clearance, Cl_H), but drugs are also metabolized in, for example, the small intestine, lungs, kidneys, and skin. In general, hydrophilic drugs of low molecular weight are excreted more easily in urine compared with large lipophilic drugs. Lipophilic and poorly water-soluble drugs are mainly metabolized and excreted in urine as hydrophilic low-molecular-weight metabolites. The total body clearance (Cl_T) is:

$$Cl_T = \frac{\text{rate of elimination}}{\text{plasma concentration}} = \frac{dD_E/dt}{C_P} = \frac{-dD_B/dt}{C_P} = \frac{k \cdot V_D \cdot C_P}{C_P} = k \cdot V_D$$

(2.95)

where, according to Eq. (2.1), $dD_B/dt = -k \cdot D_B = -k \cdot V_D \cdot C_P$ and according to Eq. (2.8) $Cl_T = V_D \cdot k$.

EXAMPLE 2.12 Total Body Clearance

A drug has $t_{\frac{1}{2}}$ of 5 h and V_D of 0.4 l/kg. What is the total body clearance of the drug in a 70-kg individual?

Answer

$$Cl_T = k \cdot V_D = \frac{\ln 2}{t_{\frac{1}{2}}} \cdot V_D = \frac{\ln 2}{5\,h} \cdot 0.4\,l/kg \cdot 70\,kg = 3.9\,l/h = 65\,ml/min$$

The *elimination rate constant* (k) is composed of several first-order rate constants, one for the renal excretion (k_e) of unmetabolized drug, one for drug metabolism in the liver (k_m), one for biliary excretion (k_b), and so on:

$$k = k_e + k_m + k_b + \cdots$$

(2.96)

and according to Eqs. (2.9) and (2.10):

$$Cl_T = V_D \cdot k_e + V_D \cdot k_m + V_D \cdot k_b + \cdots = Cl_R + Cl_H + Cl_B + \cdots = Cl_R + Cl_{NR}$$

(2.97)

where Cl_{NR} is the nonrenal clearance, including, but not limited to, Cl_H and Cl_B. Previously, we have also shown (Eq. (2.14)) that:

$$Cl_T = k \cdot V_D = \frac{F \cdot D_0}{[AUC]_0^\infty}$$

(2.98)

where F is the absolute drug availability, which is equal to unity for IV bolus injection.

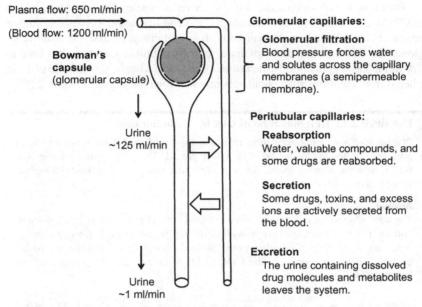

Plasma flow: 650 ml/min

(Blood flow: 1200 ml/min)

Bowman's capsule
(glomerular capsule)

Urine
~125 ml/min

Urine
~1 ml/min

Glomerular capillaries:

Glomerular filtration
Blood pressure forces water and solutes across the capillary membranes (a semipermeable membrane).

Peritubular capillaries:

Reabsorption
Water, valuable compounds, and some drugs are reabsorbed.

Secretion
Some drugs, toxins, and excess ions are actively secreted from the blood.

Excretion
The urine containing dissolved drug molecules and metabolites leaves the system.

FIGURE 2.29 Schematic representation of a nephron, the basic functional unit of the kidney. In humans, a normal kidney contains up to1.5 million nephrons. The renal blood flow is approximately 1,200 ml/min (or 650 ml plasma/min), and the total urine production is approximately 1 ml/min.

In the kidneys, drugs are excreted by glomerular filtration and by active secretion in the peritubular capillaries (Figure 2.29). Drugs excreted by glomerular filtration may be passively reabsorbed in the peritubular capillaries. Only unbound hydrophilic molecules with a molecular weight below approximately 25 kDa are filtered through glomerulus. In humans, dextrans of less than 15 kDa are mainly excreted unchanged in urine, with a renal clearance close to the GFR, whereas dextrans above about 50 kDa are mainly degraded in the liver to lower-molecular-weight products before being excreted from the body [10]. The influence of protein binding on active drug secretion depends on the efficiency of the secretion process. If the secretion of a drug is not very efficient, protein binding may decrease the secretion. However, some drugs are such excellent substrates for the secretory system that they are virtually completely removed from the blood flow even when they are bound to plasma proteins. Renal clearance is:

$$Cl_R = \frac{\text{rate of excretion}}{\text{plasma concentration}} = \frac{\text{filtration rate} + \text{secretion rate} - \text{reabsorption rate}}{C_P}$$

$$= \frac{dD_U/dt}{C_P}$$

(2.99)

Inulin is a polysaccharide, with an average molecular weight of about 5,000 Da, consisting of $\beta(2,1)$-linked glucosyl and fructosyl moieties that cannot be metabolized within the human body. It is eliminated unchanged in urine by glomerular filtration and does not undergo reabsorption or secretion. It is used to determine kidney function by determining the GFR, that is, the volume of fluid filtered from the glomerular capillaries into the Bowman capsule (Figure 2.29).

EXAMPLE 2.13 Determination of GFR by Inulin Infusion

Plasma inulin concentration was maintained at 0.01 mg/ml by constant inulin infusion. Urine was collected over a 5-h period. The total urine volume was 0.65 l, and the urinary inulin concentration was determined to be 0.48 mg/ml. What is the GFR?

Answer

The total amount of inulin eliminated (dD_E/dt) was 312 mg in 5 h, or 62.4 mg/h, and the plasma inulin concentration (C_P) during the 5-h period was 0.01 mg/ml. Since inulin is only eliminated from the body by glomerular filtration, inulin clearance (Cl_{inulin}) is equal to the GFR, and thus we can use Eq. (2.99) to calculate the GFR:

$$GFR = Cl_{inulin} = \frac{\text{rate of elimination}}{\text{plasma concentration}} = \frac{dD_E/dt}{C_P} = \frac{62.4\ \text{mg}/h}{0.01\ \text{mg}/ml} = 6,240\ \text{ml}/h$$

$$= 104\ \text{ml}/\text{min}$$

Although determination of the GFR by inulin is considered one of the best methods to access renal function, it is seldom used in clinical testing, since it is somewhat complicated as well as time consuming. The more common method to access renal function is determination of the *creatinine clearance* (Cl_{cr}). Creatinine is a degradation product of creatine phosphate in muscle and is produced at a fairly constant rate. Creatinine is eliminated from the body by glomerular filtration, although a small amount is also eliminated by tubular secretion; thus, GFR estimated by Cl_{cr} tends to be higher than that determined by Cl_{inulin}. Since creatine production is proportional to muscle mass, it varies with age, weight, and gender. If the rates of urinary excretion of creatine and the plasma or serum creatine concentration (C_{cr}) are known, Cl_{cr} can be calculated from Eq. (2.99). In children (before puberty), the following equation can be used to estimate Cl_{cr} [11]:

$$Cl_{cr} = \frac{0.55 \cdot \text{body length in cm}}{C_{cr}} \tag{2.100}$$

In adult males, the following equation can be used [12]:

$$Cl_{cr} = \frac{[140 - \text{age(years)}] \cdot \text{body weight(kg)}}{72 \cdot C_{cr}(\text{mg}/100\ \text{ml})} \tag{2.101}$$

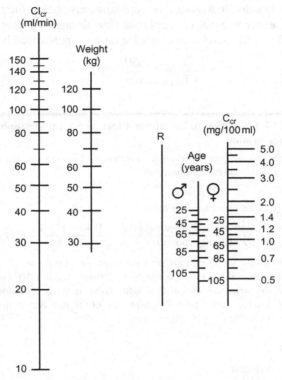

FIGURE 2.30 Nomogram for evaluation of creatine clearance (Cl_{cr}) from weight, gender, and C_{cr}. The nomogram is used as follows. (1) A line is drawn connecting the person's weight and age. (2) Then, a line drawn from the person's C_{cr} through the R intersection of line 1 and Cl_{cr} is read from the axis intercept furthest to the left [13].

In females, Eq. (2.101) is used, but the value obtained is multiplied by 0.90. Alternatively, the nomogram in Figure 2.30 can be used.

According to Eq. (2.99), Cl_R is the sum of the GFR and active tubular secretion rate, less the tubular reabsorption rate, divided by the plasma concentration; for inulin, $Cl_T = Cl_R = GFR$. Since inulin is cleared completely by the kidneys and only by glomerular filtration, the clearance ratio (Cl_{drug}/Cl_{inulin}) may give an indication of how a given drug is renally excreted.

Clearance ratio	Possible explanation
$\dfrac{Cl_{drug}}{Cl_{inulin}} > 1$	Glomerular filtration and tubular excretion
$\dfrac{Cl_{drug}}{Cl_{inulin}} = 1$	Glomerular filtration only
$\dfrac{Cl_{drug}}{Cl_{inulin}} < 1$	1. Drug protein binding 2. Tubular reabsorption 3. Very large V_D (possibly due to tissue binding)

Cl_{inulin} in healthy individuals is approximately 125 ml/min. Maximum drug renal clearance is equal to the plasma flow through the kidneys or about 650 ml/min. Thus, the maximum clearance ratio is approximately:

$$\frac{Cl_{drug}}{Cl_{inulin}} \approx \frac{650}{125} = 5.2$$

EXAMPLE 2.14 Estimation of Creatinine Clearance from Creatinine Plasma Concentration

The serum creatinine concentration in a woman (25 years, 70 kg) was determined to be 3.0 mg/100 ml. Estimate her Cl_{Cr}.

Answer
From Eq. (2.101), we can calculate that:

$$Cl_{cr} = \frac{[140 - age(years)] \cdot body\ weight(kg)}{72 \cdot C_{cr}(mg/100\ ml)} = \frac{[140 - 25] \cdot 70}{72 \cdot 3.0} = 37\ ml/min$$

For a male, it would be 37 ml/min, and for a female, it will be 37 × 0.90, or 33 ml/min. Alternatively, we can estimate Cl_{Cr} from Figure 2.30. First, draw a line between the woman's age and weight. Then, draw a new line from the determined C_{Cr} value through the R-intersection of the first line to the Cl_{Cr} axis, and read the Cl_{Cr} value ($Cl_{Cr} \approx 30$ ml/min):

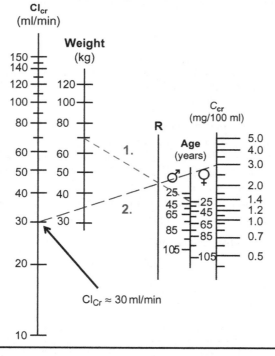

EXAMPLE 2.15 *p*-Aminohippuric Acid and Active Tubular Secretion

p-Aminohippuric acid (PAH) was used to measure active tubular secretion in a male with normal Cl_{Cr}. Plasma flowing through the kidneys is completely cleared of PAH, and thus PAH is commonly used to determine active tubular secretion. The plasma concentration of PAH was maintained at 0.01 mg/ml by IV infusion, and 19.5 mg of PAH was eliminated unchanged in urine during a 3-min collection period. Calculate Cl_R for PAH, and determine the renal blood flow.

Answer
From Eq. (2.99), we can calculate that:

$$Cl_R = \frac{dD_U/dt}{C_P} = \frac{19.5 \text{ mg/3 min}}{0.01 \text{ mg/ml}} = 650 \text{ ml/min}$$

The Cl_R of PAH is determined to be 650 ml/min, and thus the plasma flow through the kidneys (Q_{plasma}) is 650 ml/min, corresponding to a blood flow of 1,200 ml/min (see Figure 2.29).

Note that like most active processes in the human body, active tubular PAH secretion can become saturated at very high PAH plasma concentrations.

Hepatic clearance (Cl_H) results from drug biotransformation (metabolism) in the liver and biliary excretion of unmetabolized drug, although biliary excretion of unchanged drug is frequently referred to as *biliary clearance* (Cl_B). Each metabolite (e.g., A, B, and C, etc.) has its own first-order rate constant, and thus it is possible to extend Eq. (2.96):

$$k = k_e + k_m + k_b + \cdots = k_e + k_{m_A} + k_{m_B} + k_{m_C} + k_b + \cdots \qquad (2.102)$$

However, for simplicity, we assume that $k = k_e + k_m$ and $Cl_T = Cl_R + Cl_H$, or $Cl_T = Cl_R + Cl_{NR}$, unless otherwise indicated. The hepatic clearance is the volume of blood entering the liver that is cleared of the drug per unit time (Figure 2.31):

$$Cl_H = \frac{Q \cdot (C_A - C_V)}{C_A} = Q \cdot ER \qquad (2.103)$$

The liver extraction ratio (ER) is a measure of drug removal by the liver after oral administration:

$$ER = \frac{(C_A - C_V)}{C_A} \qquad (2.104)$$

Since protein bound drug molecules are practically unable to permeate biologic membranes or bind to enzymes, drug protein binding can protect drugs against metabolism. Thus, Cl_H is frequently proportional to the fraction of unbound drug (f_u). This is especially true for drugs with low ER (<0.3), for example, diazepam, theophylline, and warfarin. However, drugs

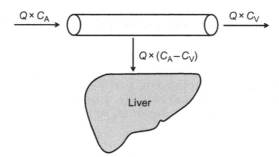

FIGURE 2.31 Schematic explanation of hepatic clearance. Q is the blood flow through the liver, C_A is the drug concentration in the blood entering the liver via the portal vein, and C_V is the drug concentration in the blood leaving the liver.

with high ER (>0.7), for example, lidocaine, propranolol, and verapamil, are extensively cleared from the blood flow by the liver, and thus their protein binding has little effect on their Cl_H. Their Cl_H depends mainly on hepatic blood flow (Q in Figure 2.31). Then, there are drugs with intermediate ER, whose Cl_H is dependent on both Q and f_u as well as on the intrinsic capacity of the liver to metabolize the drug.

EXAMPLE 2.16 Hepatic Clearance of Verapamil

Verapamil, a calcium channel blocker, is used to treat high blood pressure and certain abnormal heart rhythms and is commonly prescribed to patients with congestive heart failure. The half-life ($t_{1/2}$) of verapamil is 4 h, the apparent volume of distribution (V_D) is 4 l/kg. Verapamil is 90% plasma protein bound, and less than 3% of the drug is excreted unchanged in urine.

A. Calculate the hepatic clearance of verapamil in an adult male patient (62 years old; 105 kg) ignoring urinary excretion.

B. Estimate the ER for verapamil if the hepatic blood flow (Q) is assumed to be 1,500 ml/min.

C. How would hepatic diseases such as cirrhosis affect the oral absorption and Cl_H of verapamil?

D. How will decreased protein binding affect Cl_H of verapamil?

E. What is a first-pass effect?

F. Bioavailability of a new verapamil tablet was tested and shown that the relative availability (F_{rel}) of the tablet, compared with that of oral solution, was 80% and that the absolute availability (F) of the tablet was 16%. Determine the relative and absolute availability of the verapamil tablet. Is it possible to improve the absolute availability of the tablet through reformulation?

Answer

A. $V_D = 4 l/kg \times 105\ kg = 420\ l$ $k = \dfrac{\ln 2}{t_{1/2}} = \dfrac{0.693}{4\ h} = 0.173\ h^{-1}$

$Cl_H = V_D \cdot k = 420\ l \cdot 0.173\ h^{-1} = 72.7\ l\ h^{-1} = 1{,}210\ ml/min$

B. $Cl_H = Q \cdot ER \Rightarrow ER = \frac{Cl_H}{Q} = \frac{1,210 \text{ ml/min}}{1,500 \text{ ml/min}} = 0.8$

C. Hepatic diseases such as cirrhosis will reduce Cl_H. Verapamil undergoes extensive first-pass effect, and decreased Cl_H will result in decreased ER. This will decrease the first-pass effect, which leads to increased F.

D. Since verapamil has relatively high ER, decreased protein binding will have insignificant effect on Cl_H.

E. After oral absorption, the drug enters the general blood circulation via the portal vein, which carries blood from the GI tract to the liver. A drug with high ER will undergo extensive first-pass effect whereby significant amounts of the drug are removed from the blood before it reaches the systemic blood circulation.

F. Eighty percent of drug in the tablet is absorbed into the portal vein. Then the liver extracts 80% of the drug (80% of the drug in the tablet) before it reaches the systemic blood circulation. Thus, only 20% of the 80%, or 16%, of drug in the tablet reaches the systemic circulation (i.e., $F = 0.16$). In other words, the pharmaceutical availability of the tablet is 80%, but the biologic availability is only 20%. It is possible to increase F from 0.16 to 0.20 through improved formulation, but that is the maximum absolute availability that can be obtained through tablet reformulation.

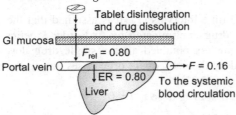

2.7 MULTIPLE-DOSE REGIMENS

Until now, only single-dose administration has been discussed, although in most cases, drugs are given in multiple doses. In a multiple-dosage regimen, C_P will rise and fall but generally C_P must be kept within the therapeutic window at all times, above the minimum effective concentration (MEC) but below the minimum toxic concentration (MTC). Some drugs have a wide therapeutic window (therapeutic index) and are easily maintained within the window, whereas others have a narrow therapeutic window (see Section 1.1) and are more difficult to administer. Multiple-dose regimen are based on pharmacokinetic parameters obtained from a single-dose administration, drug dose (D_0), and the dosage interval (τ), assuming fixed intervals between administrations.

2.7.1 Multiple-Dosage by IV Bolus Injection and One-Compartment Open Model

Mathematically, the simplest case of multiple dosage is when a drug, which is distributed according to the one-compartment open model, is administered

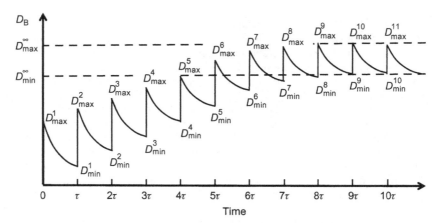

FIGURE 2.32 Schematic drawing showing the total amount of drug in the body (D_B) as a function of time. Equal drug doses (D_0) are given by IV bolus injection every τ hours. The pharmacokinetic parameters (e.g., k) remain constant during the drug treatment.

via IV bolus injection at fixed time intervals (τ). It is assumed that the drug dosages are additive, that the drug is eliminated by first-order kinetics, and that the pharmacokinetic parameters obtained after a single drug dose (the first drug dose) are not altered by the subsequent drug doses during the multidose drug administration (Figure 2.32).

After administration of the first drug dose at $t = 0$:

$$D^1_{max} = D_0$$

$$D^1_{min} = D_0 \cdot e^{-k \cdot \tau}$$

where D^1_{max} is the total maximum amount of drug in the body immediately after IV bolus administration of the first dose, and D^1_{min} is the total minimum amount of drug in the body immediately before administration of the second dose. Then, after administration of the second drug dose at $t = \tau$, we have:

$$D^2_{max} = D_0 + D^1_{min} = D_0 + D_0 \cdot e^{-k \cdot \tau} = D_0(1 + e^{-k \cdot \tau})$$

$$D^2_{min} = D^2_{max} \cdot e^{-k \cdot \tau} = D_0(1 + e^{-k \cdot \tau}) \cdot e^{-k \cdot \tau} = D_0(e^{-k \cdot \tau} + e^{-2k \cdot \tau})$$

After administration of the third drug dose at $t = 2\tau$:

$$D^3_{max} = D_0 + D^2_{min} = D_0 + D_0(e^{-k \cdot \tau} + e^{-2k \cdot \tau}) = D_0(1 + e^{-k \cdot \tau} + e^{-2k \cdot \tau})$$

$$D^3_{min} = D^3_{max} \cdot e^{-k \cdot \tau} = D_0(1 + e^{-k \cdot \tau} + e^{-2k \cdot \tau}) \cdot e^{-k \cdot \tau} = D_0(e^{-k \cdot \tau} + e^{-2k \cdot \tau} + e^{-3k \cdot \tau})$$

After administration of the fourth drug dose at $t = 3\tau$:

$$D^3_{max} = D_0 + D^2_{min} = D_0(1 + e^{-k \cdot \tau} + e^{-2k \cdot \tau} + e^{-3k \cdot \tau})$$

$$D_{min}^3 = D_{max}^3 \cdot e^{-k \cdot \tau} = D_0(e^{-k \cdot \tau} + e^{-2k \cdot \tau} + e^{-3k \cdot \tau} + e^{-4k \cdot \tau})$$

After administration of the *n*th dose at $t = (n - 1)\tau$:

$$D_{max}^n = D_0(1 + e^{-k \cdot \tau} + e^{-2k \cdot \tau} + \cdots + e^{-(n-1) \cdot k \cdot \tau})$$

$$D_{min}^n = D_{max}^n \cdot e^{-k \cdot \tau} = D_0(e^{-k \cdot \tau} + e^{-2k \cdot \tau} + e^{-3k \cdot \tau} + \cdots + e^{-nk \cdot \tau})$$

It can be seen that if $r = 1 + e^{-k \cdot \tau} + e^{-2k \cdot \tau} + \cdots + e^{-(n-1) \cdot k \cdot \tau}$, then:

$$D_{max}^n = D_0 \cdot r \tag{2.105}$$

$$D_{min}^n = D_{max}^n \cdot e^{-k \cdot \tau} = D_0 \cdot r \cdot e^{-k \cdot \tau} \tag{2.106}$$

$$r = 1 + e^{-k \cdot \tau} + e^{-2k \cdot \tau} + \cdots + e^{-(n-1) \cdot k \cdot \tau} \tag{2.107}$$

$$r \cdot e^{-k \cdot \tau} = e^{-k \cdot \tau} + e^{-2k \cdot \tau} + e^{-3k \cdot \tau} + \cdots + e^{-n \cdot k \cdot \tau} \tag{2.108}$$

Subtracting Eq. (2.108) from Eq. (2.107) gives:

$$r - r \cdot e^{-k \cdot \tau} = 1 - e^{-n \cdot k \cdot \tau} \tag{2.109}$$

Rearrangement of Eq. (2.109) gives:

$$r = \frac{1 - e^{-n \cdot k \cdot \tau}}{1 - e^{-k \cdot \tau}} \tag{2.110}$$

Substituting Eq. (2.110) into Eqs. (2.105) and (2.106) gives:

$$D_{max}^n = D_0 \cdot \left(\frac{1 - e^{-n \cdot k \cdot \tau}}{1 - e^{-k \cdot \tau}} \right) \tag{2.111}$$

$$D_{min}^n = D_0 \cdot \left(\frac{1 - e^{-n \cdot k \cdot \tau}}{1 - e^{-k \cdot \tau}} \right) \cdot e^{-k \cdot \tau} \tag{2.112}$$

$$D_B^n = D_0 \cdot \left(\frac{1 - e^{-n \cdot k \cdot \tau}}{1 - e^{-k \cdot \tau}} \right) \cdot e^{-k \cdot t} \tag{2.113}$$

where D_B^n is the total amount of drug in the body after administration of the *n*th dose, and t is the time from administration of the last dose. After drug administration for some time ($n = \infty$), we get:

$$D_{max}^\infty = D_0 \cdot \left(\frac{1}{1 - e^{-k \cdot \tau}} \right) \tag{2.114}$$

$$D_{min}^\infty = D_0 \cdot \left(\frac{1}{1 - e^{-k \cdot \tau}} \right) \cdot e^{-k \cdot \tau} \tag{2.115}$$

$$D_B^\infty = D_0 \cdot \left(\frac{1}{1 - e^{-k \cdot \tau}} \right) \cdot e^{-k \cdot t} \tag{2.116}$$

Dividing V_D into Eqs. (2.111) to (2.116) gives the corresponding equations for drug plasma concentrations:

$$C_{max}^n = \frac{D_0}{V_D} \cdot \left(\frac{1 - e^{-n \cdot k \cdot \tau}}{1 - e^{-k \cdot \tau}} \right) \tag{2.117}$$

$$C_{min}^n = \frac{D_0}{V_D} \cdot \left(\frac{1 - e^{-n \cdot k \cdot \tau}}{1 - e^{-k \cdot \tau}} \right) \cdot e^{-k \cdot \tau} \tag{2.118}$$

$$C_P^n = \frac{D_0}{V_D} \cdot \left(\frac{1 - e^{-n \cdot k \cdot \tau}}{1 - e^{-k \cdot \tau}} \right) \cdot e^{-k \cdot t} \tag{2.119}$$

$$C_{max}^{\infty} = \frac{D_0}{V_D} \cdot \left(\frac{1}{1 - e^{-k \cdot \tau}} \right) \tag{2.120}$$

$$C_{min}^{\infty} = \frac{D_0}{V_D} \cdot \left(\frac{1}{1 - e^{-k \cdot \tau}} \right) \cdot e^{-k \cdot \tau} \tag{2.121}$$

$$C_P^{\infty} = \frac{D_0}{V_D} \cdot \left(\frac{1}{1 - e^{-k \cdot \tau}} \right) \cdot e^{-k \cdot t} \tag{2.122}$$

where t is as before the time from administration of the last dose.

2.7.2   Multiple-Dosage by Oral Administration and One-Compartment Open Model

The equations for multiple oral administration are obtained by inserting Eq. (2.110) for the elimination phase and the comparable equation for the absorption phase into Eq. (2.66):

$$
\begin{aligned}
C_P &= \frac{F \cdot k_a \cdot D_0}{V_D \cdot (k_a - k)} (r \cdot e^{-k \cdot t} - r' \cdot e^{-k_a \cdot t}) \\
&= \frac{F \cdot k_a \cdot D_0}{V_D \cdot (k_a - k)} \left(\frac{1 - e^{-n \cdot k \cdot \tau}}{1 - e^{-k \cdot \tau}} \cdot e^{-k \cdot t} - \frac{1 - e^{-n \cdot k_a \cdot \tau}}{1 - e^{-k_a \cdot \tau}} \cdot e^{-k_a \cdot t} \right)
\end{aligned}
\tag{2.123}
$$

where $r' = (1 - e^{-n \cdot k_a \cdot \tau})/(1 - e^{-k_a \cdot \tau})$. At steady-state, where $n = \infty$, the following equation is obtained, where t is the time from administration of the last dose:

$$C_P^{\infty} = \frac{F \cdot k_a \cdot D_0}{V_D \cdot (k_a - k)} \left(\frac{1}{1 - e^{-k \cdot \tau}} \cdot e^{-k \cdot t} - \frac{1}{1 - e^{-k_a \cdot \tau}} \cdot e^{-k_a \cdot t} \right) \tag{2.124}$$

$$C_{min}^{\infty} = \frac{F \cdot k_a \cdot D_0}{V_D \cdot (k_a - k)} \left(\frac{1}{1 - e^{-k \cdot \tau}} \cdot e^{-k \cdot \tau} - \frac{1}{1 - e^{-k_a \cdot \tau}} \cdot e^{-k_a \cdot \tau} \right) \tag{2.125}$$

However, to calculate C_{max}^{∞}, we will first have to calculate the time from last drug administration to the maximum plasma concentration. t_{max} after the *first dose* is given by Eq. (2.69).

The time from drug administration to C_{max} of the subsequent doses is obtained from Eq. (2.124), keeping in mind that $dC_P^{\infty}/dt = 0$ at t_p (Figure 2.18):

$$t_p = \frac{1}{k_a - k} \cdot \ln\left[\frac{k_a(1 - e^{-k \cdot \tau})}{k(1 - e^{-k_a \cdot \tau})}\right] \tag{2.126}$$

After the first dose, C_{max} of subsequent oral doses can be obtained by substituting t_p into Eq. (2.124).

EXAMPLE 2.17 Multiple Oral Dosage of Amoxicillin

In Example 2.7, the rate constants (i.e., k_a and k) as well as t_{max} and C_{max} were determined after administration of one 500 mg amoxicillin tablet:

$$k_a = 1.10 \text{ h}^{-1}; \ k = 0.67 \text{ h}^{-1}$$

$$t_{max} = \frac{\ln(k_a/k)}{k_a - k} = \frac{\ln(1.10/0.67)}{1.10 - 0.67} = 1.2 \text{ h}$$

$$C_{max} = \frac{F \cdot k_a \cdot D_0}{V_D \cdot (k_a - k)}(e^{-k \cdot t_{max}} - e^{-k_a \cdot t_{max}}) = e^{3.51} \cdot (e^{-0.67 \cdot 1.2} - e^{-1.10 \cdot 1.2}) = 6.0 \ \mu g/ml$$

On the basis of these values, calculate C_{max}^{∞}, C_{min}^{∞} and t_p when 500 mg amoxicillin tablets are given three times per day (Latin: *ter in die*; [tid]) to the same healthy male volunteer.

Answer

We assume that the pharmacokinetics after a single drug dose (the first drug dose) are not altered by the following drug doses during the multidose drug administration. Here, $\tau = 8$ h, and t_p is calculated according to Eq. (2.126):

$$t_p = \frac{1}{k_a - k} \cdot \ln\left[\frac{k_a(1 - e^{-k \cdot \tau})}{k(1 - e^{-k_a \cdot \tau})}\right] = \frac{1}{1.10 - 0.67} \cdot \ln\left[\frac{1.10(1 - e^{-0.67 \cdot 8})}{0.67(1 - e^{-1.10 \cdot 8})}\right]$$

$$t_p = 2.33 \text{ h} \cdot \ln\left[\frac{1.10 \cdot 0.995}{0.67 \cdot 1.000}\right] = 1.1 \text{ h}$$

In Example 2.7, we determine that $(F \cdot k_a \cdot D_0)/(V_D \cdot (k_a - k)) = e^{3.5104} = 33.46 \ \mu g/ml$. C_{max}^{∞} is calculated from Eq. (2.124), where $\tau = 8$ h and $t = t_p = 1.1$ h:

$$C_{max}^{\infty} = 33.46\left(\frac{1}{1 - e^{-0.67 \cdot 8}} \cdot e^{-0.67 \cdot 1.1} - \frac{1}{1 - e^{-1.10 \cdot 8}} \cdot e^{-1.10 \cdot 1.1}\right)$$

$$= 33.46 \cdot (0.48 - 0.30) = 6.0 \ \mu g/ml$$

C_{min}^{∞} is calculated from Eq. (2.125):

$$C_{min}^{\infty} = \frac{F \cdot k_a \cdot D_0}{V_D \cdot (k_a - k)} \left(\frac{1}{1 - e^{-k \cdot \tau}} \cdot e^{-k \cdot \tau} - \frac{1}{1 - e^{-k_a \cdot \tau}} \cdot e^{-k_a \cdot \tau} \right)$$

$$= 33.46 \left(\frac{e^{-0.67 \cdot 8}}{1 - e^{-0.67 \cdot 8}} - \frac{e^{-1.10 \cdot 8}}{1 - e^{-1.10 \cdot 8}} \right) = 33.46 \cdot 0.0045 = 0.15 \ \mu g/ml$$

The $t_{\frac{1}{2}}$ of amoxicillin is only 1.0 h and, thus, there are eight half-lives between drug doses ($\tau = 8 \cdot t_{\frac{1}{2}}$). Due to this very short half-life, a very small amount of the drug is left in the body at $t = 8$ h, and consequently, $t_{max} \approx t_p$, $C_{max}^1 \approx C_{max}^{\infty}$ and $C_{min}^1 \approx C_{min}^{\infty}$.

If the half-life of the drug had been eight times longer ($t_{\frac{1}{2}} = 8$ h) but everything else were identical (including $(F \cdot k_a \cdot D_0)/(V_D \cdot (k_a - k)) = 33.46 \ \mu g/ml$), then the following values would have been obtained: $t_{max} = 2.5$ h, $t_p = 1.8$ h, $C_{max}^1 = 25 \ \mu g/ml$, $C_{max}^{\infty} = 53 \ \mu g/ml$, $C_{min}^1 = 17 \ \mu g/ml$ and $C_{min}^{\infty} = 33 \ \mu g/ml$.

2.7.3 Loading Dose

Following multiple drug dosing, in which equal drug doses are given every τ hours, the plasma levels will gradually increase until steady-state has been reached, at which time the amount of drug eliminated from the body between drug dosing equals the drug dose (Figure 2.32). After parenteral bolus administration, the fraction of steady-state (f_{ss}) can be calculated by dividing Eq. (2.119) by Eq. (2.122):

$$f_{ss} = \frac{C_P^n}{C_P^{\infty}} = \frac{(D_0/V_D) \cdot ((1 - e^{-n \cdot k \cdot \tau})/(1 - e^{-k \cdot \tau})) \cdot e^{-k \cdot t}}{(D_0/V_D) \cdot (1/(1 - e^{-k \cdot \tau})) \cdot e^{-k \cdot t}} = 1 - e^{-n \cdot k \cdot \tau} \tag{2.127}$$

The time ($n \cdot \tau$) it takes to reach some given fraction of steady-state (f_{ss}) can be calculated by the following equation that is derived from Eq. (2.127):

$$n \cdot t = \frac{\ln(1 - f_{ss})}{-k} = \frac{\ln(1 - f_{ss})}{-0.693} \cdot t_{\frac{1}{2}} \tag{2.128}$$

Equation (2.128) shows that it takes one $t_{\frac{1}{2}}$ to reach 50% of steady-state (i.e., $f_{ss} = 0.50$), 3.32 $t_{\frac{1}{2}}$ to reach 90% of steady-state, 6.64 $t_{\frac{1}{2}}$ to reach 99% of steady-state and 10 $t_{\frac{1}{2}}$ to reach 99.9% of steady-state (Figure 2.33). Likewise after oral administration the following equation is obtained:

$$f_{ss} = \frac{C_P^n}{C_P^{\infty}} = 1 + \frac{k \cdot e^{-n \cdot k_a \cdot \tau}}{k_a - k} - \frac{k_a \cdot e^{-n \cdot k \cdot \tau}}{k_a - k} \tag{2.129}$$

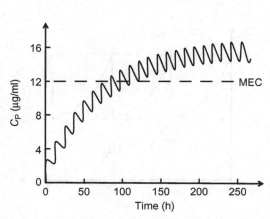

FIGURE 2.33 Sketch showing the plasma concentration after oral administration of a hypo-thetical drug with MEC of $12\,\mu g/ml$ ($D_0 = 100$ mg, $\tau = 12$ h, $F = 1.00$, $t_{\frac{1}{2}} = 50$ h, $V_D = 38$ l).

If k_a/k is10 or greater, then the absorption phase can be ignored, and Eq. (2.128) can be used for multiple oral dosage.

For the drug in Figure 2.33, the therapeutic effect would not be observed until after dosing for over two half-lives or 4−5 days after administration of the first dose. To reach MEC, or therapeutic plasma levels from the beginning of a multiple drug dosing, a higher drug dose, a loading dose (D_L), is given at the beginning of the drug treatment, and that is followed by a lower maintenance dose (D_0). Sometimes, D_M is used as the symbol for maintenance dose.

For IV infusion, a loading dose is calculated according to Eq. (2.24) and given by IV bolus injection at the start of drug infusion (Figure 2.6). Equation (2.24) can also be used to calculate D_L when the drug treatment consists of multiple IV injections, that is, by multiplying the desired drug plasma concentration by V_D. Then, the maintenance dose (D_0) is the amount of drug that is eliminated from the body between doses (Figure 2.34):

$$D_0 = D_L - D_{\min}^{\infty} = D_L - D_L \cdot e^{-k \cdot \tau} \qquad (2.130)$$

Rearranging Eq. (2.130) gives:

$$\frac{D_L}{D_0} = \frac{1}{1 - e^{-k \cdot \tau}} \qquad (2.131)$$

For a multiple dosing of an orally administrated drug, D_L can be calculated as follows:

$$\frac{D_L}{D_0} = \frac{1}{(1 - e^{-k_a \cdot \tau}) \cdot (1 - e^{-k \cdot \tau})} \qquad (2.132)$$

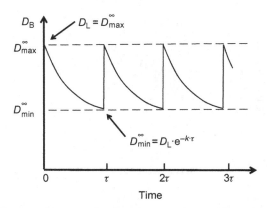

FIGURE 2.34 Concentration curve for drug dosage regimen with equal maintenance doses (D_0) and dosage intervals (τ) and a loading dose (D_L).

Another equation for rapid estimation of D_L for an orally administered drug is:

$$D_L = \frac{V_D \cdot C_{av}^{\infty}}{S \cdot F} \tag{2.133}$$

where C_{av}^{∞} is the desired average plasma drug concentration, and S is the salt form correction factor (for a basic drug S is the molecular weight of the free base divided by the molecular weight of the salt). The rule of thumb for a simple dosage regimen is to set $\tau \approx t_{1/2}$ and $D_L = 2 \cdot D_0$. These equations are all based on the one-compartment open model.

If $C_{max}^{\infty} \approx C_{max}^{1}$, then drug accumulation is insignificant, and it will not be necessary to administer a loading dose. However, if $C_{max}^{\infty} >> C_{max}^{1}$, the accumulation is significant, and administration of a loading dose should be considered. The accumulation increases with increasing $t_{1/2}$ but decreases with increasing τ:

$$\text{Accumulation} = \frac{C_{max}^{\infty}}{C_{max}^{1}} = \frac{1}{1 - e^{-k \cdot \tau}} \tag{2.134}$$

Once steady-state has been reached, C_P will fluctuate between C_{max}^{∞} and C_{min}^{∞}. For safety reasons, C_{max}^{∞} has to remain below MTC, and C_{min}^{∞} should remain above MEC. Fluctuation in C_P can be minimized by frequent administration of small doses, and no fluctuation is observed when a drug is administered via IV infusion (Figure 2.35). Likewise, the fluctuation can be reduced by sustained drug delivery, for example, by administering the drug as a sustained-release tablet.

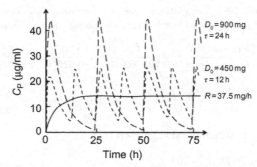

FIGURE 2.35 Sketch showing C_P–time profile after multiple oral dosing and IV infusion for a hypothetical drug ($t_{1/2} = 4$ h, $V_D = 15$ l, $F = 1.0$). The daily dose is identical (900 mg/day) for all three dosage regimens.

The average plasma concentration (Eq. (2.135)) is the same for all the profiles shown in Figure 2.35, or 14 µg/ml:

$$C_{av}^{\infty} = \frac{F \cdot D_0}{V_D \cdot k \cdot \tau} \tag{2.135}$$

EXAMPLE 2.18 Determination of an Oral Dosage Regimen for a New Drug

The following pharmacokinetic parameters for a new drug were determined in healthy volunteers: $k_a = 0.70$ h^{-1}, $k = 2.8 \times 10^{-2}$ h^{-1}, $V_D = 0.70$ l/kg, $F = 0.50$, therapeutic range 1.0 to 3.0 µg/ml, and MTL 5.0 µg/ml.

Propose a dosage regimen for multiple oral dosing of the drug for a 70-kg male.

Answer

We start by calculating the maximum time that can elapse between drug administrations by determining the time it takes for C_P to decrease from 3.0 to 1.0 µg/ml. This is done by dividing Eq. (2.118) by Eq. (2.121):

$$\frac{C_{max}^{\infty}}{C_{min}^{\infty}} = \frac{(D_0/V_D) \cdot (1/(1 - e^{-k \cdot \tau}))}{(D_0/V_D) \cdot (1/(1 - e^{-k \cdot \tau})) \cdot e^{-k \cdot \tau}} = e^{k \cdot \tau} \tag{2.136}$$

$$\frac{3.0}{1.0} = e^{0.028 \cdot \tau} \Rightarrow \tau = 39 \text{ h}$$

It takes 39 h for C_P to decrease from 3.0 to 1.0 µg/ml. Consequently, τ can be 24 h, 12 h, 8 h, or even 6 h, keeping in mind that C_P fluctuation decreases with decreasing τ. If we set $\tau = 12$ h, then we can calculate D_0 by using Eq. (2.135) and set $C_{av}^{\infty} = 2.0$ µg/ml $= 2.0$ mg/l, that is, right in the middle of therapeutic range:

$$C_{av}^{\infty} = \frac{F \cdot D_0}{V_D \cdot k \cdot \tau} \Rightarrow D_0 = \frac{C_{av}^{\infty} \cdot V_D \cdot k \cdot \tau}{F}$$

$$= \frac{2.0 \text{ mg/l} \cdot 0.70 \text{ l/kg } 70 \text{ kg} \cdot 0.028 \text{ h}^{-1} \cdot 12 \text{ h}}{0.50} = 65.85 \text{ mg}$$

On the basis of these calculations, we set the following dosage regimen: $D_0 = 70$ mg and $\tau = 12$ h, and then we test it by using Eqs. (2.126) and (2.124):

$$t_p = \frac{1}{k_a - k} \cdot \ln\left[\frac{k_a(1 - e^{-k \cdot \tau})}{k(1 - e^{-k_a \cdot \tau})}\right] = \frac{1}{0.70 - 0.028} \cdot \ln\left[\frac{0.70(1 - e^{-0.028 \cdot 12})}{0.028(1 - e^{-0.70 \cdot 12})}\right] = 2.92 \text{ h}$$

$$C_p^\infty = \frac{F \cdot k_a \cdot D_0}{V_D \cdot (k_a - k)} \left(\frac{1}{1 - e^{-k \cdot \tau}} \cdot e^{-k \cdot t} - \frac{1}{1 - e^{-k_a \cdot \tau}} \cdot e^{-k_a \cdot t}\right)$$

C_{max}^∞ when $t = t_p$ (2.30 µg/ml) and C_{min}^∞ when $t = \tau$.

$$C_{min}^\infty = \frac{0.50 \cdot 0.70 \text{ h}^{-1} \cdot 70 \text{ mg}}{0.70 \text{ } l/\text{kg} \cdot 70 \text{ kg}(0.70 - 0.028) \text{ } h^{-1}}$$
$$\left(\frac{1}{1 - e^{-0.028 \text{ h}^{-1} \cdot 12 \text{ h}}} \cdot e^{-0.028 \text{ h}^{-1} \cdot 12 \text{ h}} - \frac{1}{1 - e^{-0.70 \text{ h}^{-1} \cdot 12 \text{ h}}} \cdot e^{-0.70 \text{ h}^{-1} \cdot 12 \text{ h}}\right)$$
$$= 1.86 \text{ µg/ml}$$

Both C_{max}^∞ and C_{min}^∞ are well within the therapeutic range of 3.0–1.0 µg/ml and well below MTL of 5.0 µg/ml. According to Eq. (2.134), the accumulation is:

$$\text{Accumulation} = \frac{C_{max}^\infty}{C_{max}^1} = \frac{1}{1 - e^{-k \cdot \tau}} = \frac{1}{1 - e^{-0.028 \cdot 12}} = 3.50$$

The half-life of the drug is about 24 h and according to Eq. (2.128), it will take more than 3 days for C_P to reach 90% of steady-state. Consequently, a loading dose should be given (Eq. (2.132)):

$$D_L = \frac{70 \text{ mg}}{(1 - e^{-0.70 \cdot 12}) \cdot (1 - e^{-0.028 \cdot 12})} = \frac{70 \text{ mg}}{0.9998 \cdot 0.2854} = 245 \text{ mg}$$

Thus, the proposed dosage regimen for the drug could be $D_0 = 70$ mg, $D_L = 3 \times 70$ mg, or 210 mg and $\tau = 12$ h.

An alternative dosage regimen could possibly be $D_0 = 200$ mg, $D_L = 400$ mg and $\tau = 24$ h, but this would lead to greater fluctuation in C_P. Still another one could be $D_0 = 50$ mg and $\tau = 8$ h, but increased dosage frequency can lead to reduced patient compliance.

2.8 NONLINEAR PHARMACOKINETICS

Until now, simple first-order kinetics have been used to describe linear pharmacokinetics, where pharmacokinetic parameters such as $t_{1/2}$, AUC, and V_D are not affected by the drug dose; that is, the pharmacokinetic parameters are not affected by drug concentration within the body. However, many pharmacokinetic processes such as drug absorption and biotransformation involve saturable carrier-mediated systems and enzymes. Plasma protein binding of drugs can also become saturated at elevated drug concentrations, and changes in protein binding may affect V_D. Thus, drugs that follow linear pharmacokinetics at low drug doses may follow nonlinear pharmacokinetics when high drug doses are administered. In *non-linear pharmacokinetics* (sometimes referred

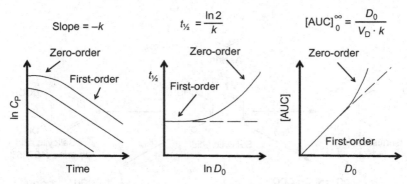

FIGURE 2.36   Sketches showing how in nonlinear pharmacokinetics, the drug dose affects the rate of drug elimination (k), $t_{1/2}$, and the AUC.

to as *dose-dependent pharmacokinetics*), the elimination rate changes from first-order to zero-order kinetics, where the apparent k decreases, and both $t_{1/2}$ and AUC increase with increasing drug dose (D_0). In nonlinear pharmacokinetics, the rate of drug elimination is capacity limited (Figure 2.36). Furthermore, nonlinear pharmacokinetics can result in increased occurrence of drug–drug interactions, when two or more drugs compete for the same enzyme. For example, in the body, aspirin is hydrolyzed to salicylic acid, which undergoes further metabolism and renal elimination. Salicylic acid is eliminated by at least five parallel routes (Figure 2.37), of which at least two (k_{m2} and k_{m4}) follow dose-dependent kinetics [14–17]. When the aspirin dose increases from about 300 mg to 10 grams (g), the salicylic acid $t_{1/2}$ increases from about 3 to 20 h due to the dose-dependent kinetics. The plasma protein binding of salicylic acid is also capacity limited and can be saturated. Consequently, not only does the observed $t_{1/2}$ of salicylic acid increase with increasing salicylic acid plasma concentration but so do the relative concentrations of the various salicylate metabolites (Figures 2.37 and 2.38).

2.8.1   Michaelis–Menten Equation

Saturable enzymatic process of drug elimination is described by Michaelis–Menten kinetics, where one enzyme (E) molecule combines with one substrate (S) molecule to form a complex (ES), which breaks down to form the product P:

$$E + S \underset{k_2}{\overset{k_1}{\rightleftharpoons}} ES \overset{k_3}{\longrightarrow} P \tag{2.137}$$

A steady-state approximation is used to solve the rate equations [18]:

$$-\frac{d[S]}{dt} = k_1[E][S] - k_2[ES] \tag{2.138}$$

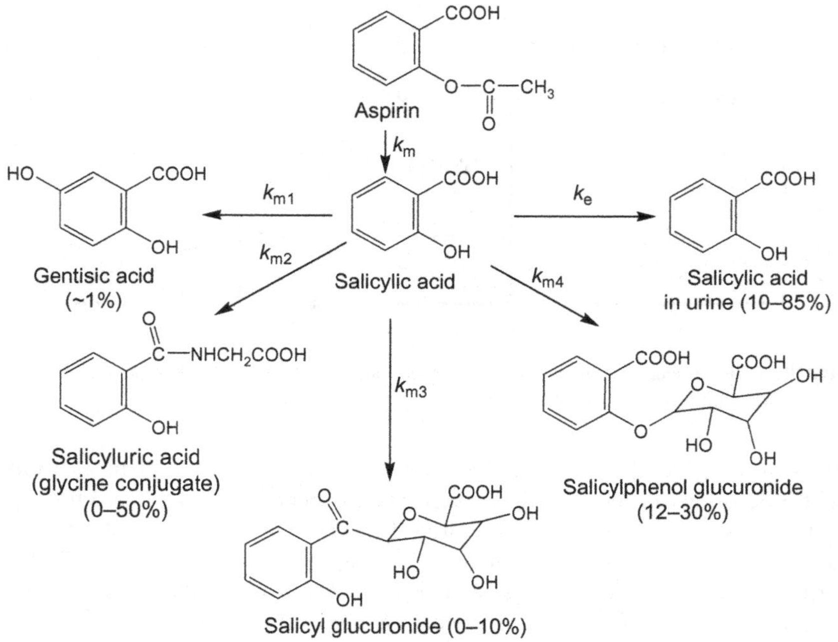

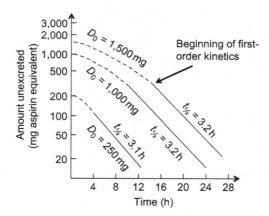

FIGURE 2.37 Metabolism and excretion of aspirin (acetylsalicylic acid), where k_e is the first-order renal excretion rate constant for renal elimination of the unchanged salicylic acid, and k_{m1} to k_{m4} are first-order rate constants for the various metabolism processes.

FIGURE 2.38 Nonlinear pharmacokinetics of salicylic acid (*broken curves*) in a male after administration of oral solution containing 250, 1,000, and 1,500 mg of aspirin. The nonlinear half-life was determined to be about 3, 7, and 8 h, respectively, but once linear kinetics was observed (*solid lines*) $t_{1/2}$ was determined to be 3.1–3.2 h [14].

$$\frac{d[ES]}{dt} = k_1[E][S] - k_2[ES] - k_3[ES] \tag{2.139}$$

$$\frac{d[P]}{dt} = k_3[ES] \tag{2.140}$$

If we assume that [ES] remains essentially constant during the course of the reaction (expressed by $[ES]_{ss}$), then Eq. (2.140) becomes:

$$\frac{d[ES]_{ss}}{dt} = k_1[E][S] - k_2[ES]_{ss} - k_3[ES]_{ss} = 0 \tag{2.141}$$

Rearrangement of Eq. (2.141) gives:

$$[ES]_{ss} = \frac{k_1[E][S]}{k_2 + k_3} \tag{2.142}$$

The total enzyme concentration ($[E]_T$) is the sum of the free (unbound) enzyme concentration ([E]) and the concentration of the enzyme–substrate complex ([ES]), or at steady-state:

$$[E]_T = [E] + [ES]_{ss} \tag{2.143}$$

Combining Eqs. (2.142) and (2.143), and rearrangement gives:

$$[ES]_{ss} = \frac{k_1[E]_T[S]}{(k_2 + k_3) + k_1[S]} \tag{2.144}$$

The *Michaelis–Menten constant* (K_m) is defined as:

$$K_m = \frac{k_2 + k_3}{k_1} \tag{2.145}$$

Combining Eqs. (2.144) and (2.145) gives:

$$[ES]_{ss} = \frac{[E]_T[S]}{K_m + [S]} \tag{2.146}$$

Combining Eqs. (2.140) and (2.146) gives the Michaelis–Menten equation:

$$\frac{d[P]}{dt} = V = k_3 \frac{[E]_T[S]}{K_m + [S]} \tag{2.147}$$

where V is the velocity (d[P]/dt). *Maximum velocity* (V_{max}) is obtained when the enzyme is saturated with the substrate (i.e., when $[ES]_{ss}$ in Eq. (2.140) is equal to $[E]_T$) and, thus, V_{max} is defined as:

$$V_{max} = k_3[E]_T \tag{2.148}$$

Combining Eqs. (2.147) and (2.148) gives the commonly observed form of Michaelis–Menten equation:

$$V = \frac{V_{max}[S]}{K_m + [S]} \tag{2.149}$$

At steady-state, the substrate disappears at the same rate as the product appears (i.e., $-d[S]/dt = d[P]/dt$) and thus:

$$-\frac{d[S]}{dt} = \frac{V_{max}[S]}{K_m + [S]} \tag{2.150}$$

In pharmacokinetics, Eq. (2.150) is more frequently written as:

$$-\frac{dC_p}{dt} = \frac{V_{max}C_P}{K_m + C_P} \tag{2.151}$$

Equations (2.150) and (2.151) can then be rearranged to obtain the values of V_{max} and K_m.

EXAMPLE 2.19 Nonlinear Elimination of a Drug

Nonlinear elimination of a drug was observed in healthy volunteers after IV bolus injection ($D_0 = 4$ g). C_P^0 was estimated to be 55 µg/ml. Calculate V_{max} and K_m from the values given in the table below:

t (min)	C_P (µg/ml)
40	38.02
70	25.51
150	2.38
165	0.93

Answer

First, we need to rearrange Eq. (2.151):

$$-\frac{dC_P}{C_P}(K_m + C_P) = V_{max}dt \tag{2.152}$$

Integration of Eq. (2.152) gives:

$$\frac{C_P^0 - C_P^t}{t} = V_{max} - \frac{K_m}{t}\ln\frac{C_P^0}{C_P^t} \tag{2.153}$$

Thus, the plot of $(C_P^0 - C_P^t)/t$ versus $\ln(C_P^0/C_P^t)/t$ will give a linear plot:

Time (min)	$C_P^0 - C_P^t$ (µg/ml)	t (min)	$\frac{C_P^0 - C_P^t}{t}$ (µg/ml/ min)	$\ln\frac{C_P^0}{C_P^t}$	$\frac{\ln(C_P^0/C_P^t)}{t}$ (min^{-1})
0–40	16.98	40	0.4245	0.3692	0.00923
40–70	29.49	70	0.4213	0.7683	0.01098
70–150	52.62	150	0.3508	3.1402	0.02093
150–165	54.07	165	0.3277	4.0799	0.02477

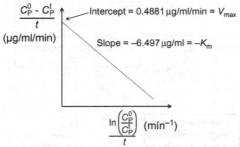

Here, $V_{max} = 0.49\ \mu g\ ml^{-1}\ min^{-1}$ and $K_m = 6.50\ \mu g/ml$.

At very low drug plasma concentration, when $C_P \ll K_m$ Eq. (2.151) approaches a first-order reaction:

$$-\frac{dC_P}{dt} = \frac{V_{max} C_P}{K_m + C_P} \approx \frac{V_{max} C_P}{K_m} = k' C_P \qquad (2.154)$$

where k' is the observed first-order rate constant. In the example above, k' is:

$$k' = \frac{0.49}{6.50} = 7.5 \times 10^{-2}\ min^{-1}$$

2.9 DRUG METABOLISM

Xenobiotics (i.e., compounds that are foreign to the body) such as drugs and pharmaceutical excipients undergo biochemical modification, that is, biotransformation or metabolism, within the body usually through specialized enzymatic systems. The liver is the main site of drug metabolism, but drug metabolizing enzymes are found in many other tissues, including the kidneys and intestinal mucosa as well as blood plasma. Drug molecules must possess some lipophilicity (as well as aqueous solubility) to be effectively absorbed from the GI tract, but only relatively hydrophilic molecules undergo renal excretion. Lipophilic drugs and excipients have to be transformed into hydrophilic metabolites that are easily excreted by the kidneys (Figure 2.39). Hydrophilic and low-molecular-weight compounds are excreted more easily from the body compared with lipophilic and high-molecular-weight compounds.

Metabolic pathways of drugs can be divided into three phases. In *phase I* (Table 2.5), polar groups are introduced into lipophilic drugs; these then can undergo conjugation in *phase II* (Table 2.6) to form more polar metabolites, which are readily excreted in urine. For example, phenytoin is practically insoluble in water. It undergoes phase I reaction, in which a hydroxyl group is introduced in position 4 on one of the two phenyl moieties to form *p*-hydroxyphenytoin (5-(4-hydroxyphenyl)-5-phenylhydantoin). Then, in a phase II reaction, the hydroxyl group serves as a substrate for the formation of an ether glucuronide (Figure 2.40). This has been reported to be the major

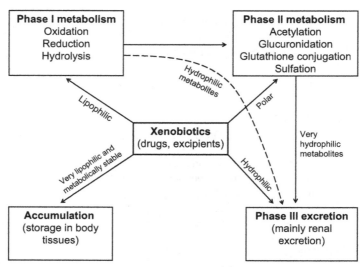

FIGURE 2.39   Schematic presentation of metabolic pathways and drug excretion. The main objectives of phase I reactions are to increase the hydrophilicity of a drug molecule and facilitate phase II conjugations. The main objectives of phase II reactions are formation of pharmacologically inactive, highly polar conjugates that are readily excreted from the body.

TABLE 2.5 Major Reactions Involved in Phase I Metabolism

	Reaction	Examples
Oxidation:		
Aromatic hydroxylation	(benzene ring → benzene ring with OH)	Phenytoin, propranolol, salicylic acid
Side chain hydroxylation	$R-CH_2CH_3 \longrightarrow R-\underset{OH}{CHCH_3}$	Cyclosporine, ibuprofen, midazolam
N-dealkylation	$R-NHCH_3 \longrightarrow R-NH_2 + CH_2O$	Diazepam, codeine, theophylline
O-dealkylation	$R-OCH_3 \longrightarrow R-OH + CH_2O$	Codeine, indomethacin
S-dealkylation	$R-SCH_3 \longrightarrow R-SH + CH_2O$	6-Methylthiopurine
Deamination	$R-\underset{NH_2}{CHCH_3} \longrightarrow R-\underset{NH_2}{\overset{OH}{CCH_3}} \longrightarrow R-\overset{O}{CCH_3} + NH_3$	Amphetamine, diazepam
N-oxidation	$\underset{R_2}{\overset{R_1}{>}}NH \longrightarrow \underset{R_2}{\overset{R_1}{>}}N-OH$	Chlorpheniramine, dapsone

(Continued)

TABLE 2.5 (Continued)

	Reaction	Examples
S-oxidation	R_1–S–R_2 $\longrightarrow$ R_1–S=O–R_2	Cimetidine, chlorpromazine, omeprazole
Reduction:		
Nitro reduction		Chloramphenicol
Reductive hydrolysis	$R–ONO_2 \longrightarrow R–OH + NO_2^-$	Nitroglycerin
Hydrolysis:		
Ester hydrolysis	R_1–C(=O)–OR_2 $\longrightarrow$ R_1–C(=O)–OH + R_2–OH	Aspirin, Enalapril, cocaine
Amide hydrolysis	R_1–C(=O)–NHR_2 $\longrightarrow$ R_1–C(=O)–OH + R_2–NH_2	Lidocaine, indomethacin

TABLE 2.6 Major Reactions Involved in Phase II Metabolism

	Reaction	Examples
Acetylation	$CoAS–C(=O)–CH_3 + RNH_2 \longrightarrow R–N–C(=O)–CH_3 + CoASH$	Isoniazid, sulfonamides
Glucuronidation		Acetaminophen, morphine, oxazepam, salicylic acid
Glutathione conjugation	RX + Cys(Glu)(Gly)–SH $\longrightarrow$ HX + Cys(Glu)(Gly)–S–R	Adriamycin, busulfan
Sulfation	$PAPS + ROH \longrightarrow R–O–S(=O)(=O)–OH + PAP$	Acetaminophen, steroids

PAPS, 3′-phosphoadenosine-5′-phosphosulfate; PAP, 3′-phosphoadenosine-5′-phosphate

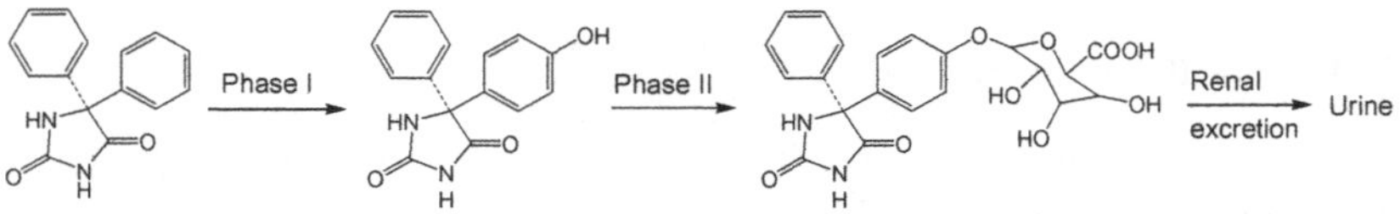

Phenytoin
insoluble in water

p-Hydroxyphenytoin
slightly soluble in water

Phenytoin ether glucuronide
highly soluble in water

FIGURE 2.40 The major metabolic pathway of phenytoin.

metabolic pathway of phenytoin in healthy subjects [19]. Some hydrophilic drugs and pharmaceutical excipients are excreted unchanged in urine, and drugs possessing polar groups in their structure may go directly to phase II (Figures 2.37 and 2.39). Metabolite formed by phase II reaction may, in some cases, undergo further metabolism before excretion (*phase III*).

In general, drug metabolites are less biologically active than the drug itself, but some metabolites are biologically active and can bind to receptors to produce pharmacologic response or side effects. Figure 2.41 shows the metabolic pathway of diazepam. The drug undergoes oxidation, hydroxylation, and glucuronidation in the liver. Several pharmacologically active metabolites such as temazepam, nordiazepam, and oxazepam are formed. Oxazepam and temazepam are conjugated with glucuronide to form highly hydrophilic glucuronides and excreted mainly in urine. Nordiazepam is the main active metabolite of diazepam. Nordiazepam has much longer $t_{1/2}$ compared with diazepam, and thus the pharmacologic activity is extended beyond diazepam elimination [20−22].

2.10 DRUG PERMEATION THROUGH BIOMEMBRANES AND DRUG TRANSPORTERS

2.10.1 Biomembranes

Biomembranes (i.e., biologic membranes) form permeation barriers within the body. The basic structure of cellular biomembranes is the lipid bilayer, composed of about 4-nanometers (nm) thick double layer of phospholipids, with occasional intertwined proteins, some of which function as channel formers, drug transporters, or drug-metabolizing enzymes (Figure 2.42). The hydrophobic tails of the two phospholipid layers face one another, whereas their hydrophilic phosphate moieties face the aqueous medium on either side of the membrane. Epithelial and endothelial membrane barriers formed by one or more layers of closely packed cells on a thin sheet of connective tissue separate the body from its environment and individual body compartments from each other. The *epithelium* is a membrane tissue that covers almost all body surfaces such as the skin, lungs, nasal cavity, buccal cavity, intestine, and other body cavities. The *endothelium* consists of thin layer of cells that lines the interior surface of blood vessels. Although similar,

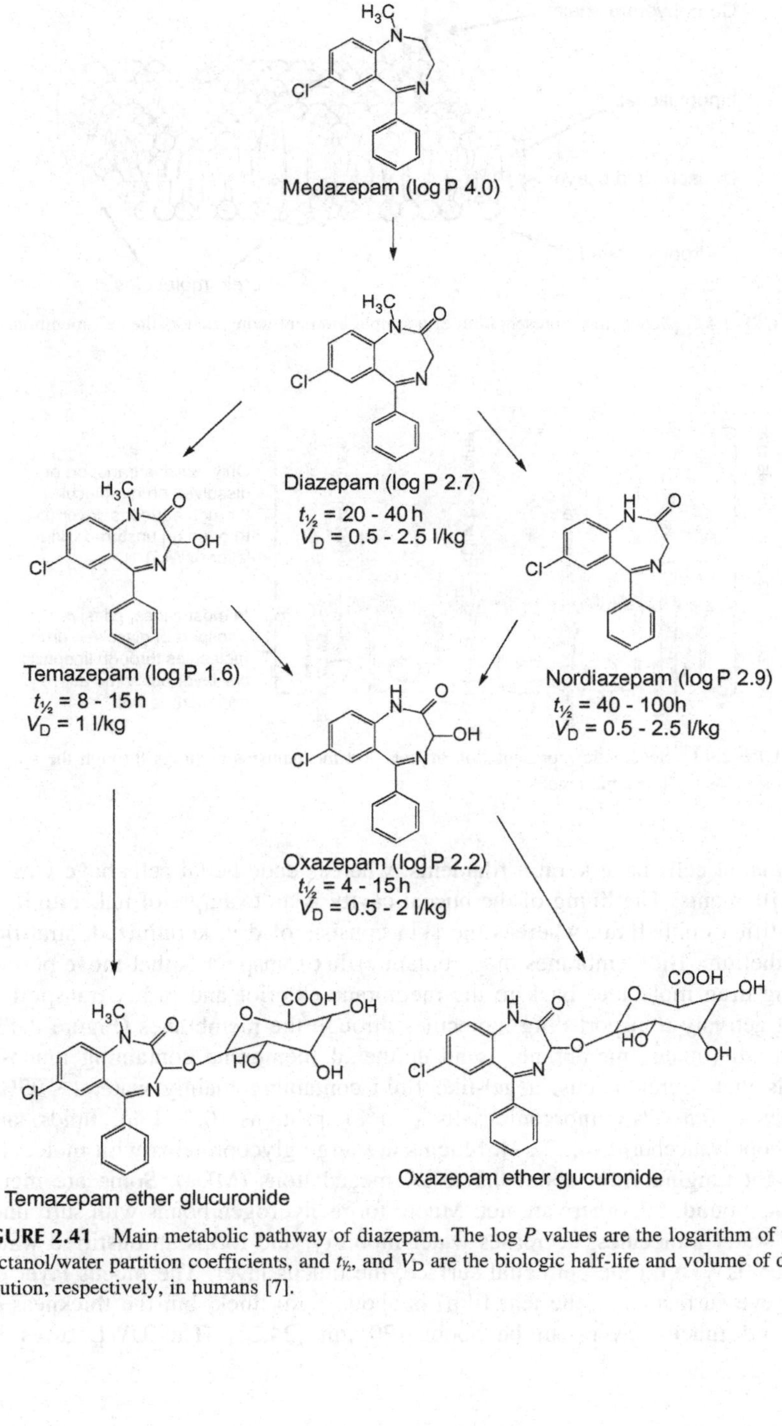

Medazepam (log P 4.0)

Diazepam (log P 2.7)
$t_{1/2}$ = 20 - 40 h
V_D = 0.5 - 2.5 l/kg

Temazepam (log P 1.6)
$t_{1/2}$ = 8 - 15 h
V_D = 1 l/kg

Nordiazepam (log P 2.9)
$t_{1/2}$ = 40 - 100h
V_D = 0.5 - 2.5 l/kg

Oxazepam (log P 2.2)
$t_{1/2}$ = 4 - 15 h
V_D = 0.5 - 2 l/kg

Temazepam ether glucuronide

Oxazepam ether glucuronide

FIGURE 2.41 Main metabolic pathway of diazepam. The log *P* values are the logarithm of the 1-octanol/water partition coefficients, and $t_{1/2}$, and V_D are the biologic half-life and volume of distribution, respectively, in humans [7].

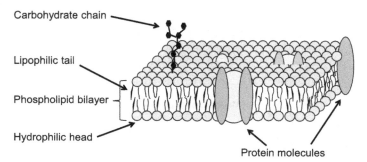

FIGURE 2.42 Schematic representation of a simple biomembrane such as the cell membrane.

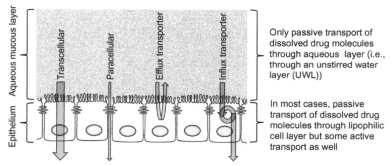

FIGURE 2.43 Schematic representation of transport mechanisms of drugs through the epithelium such as the intestinal mucosa.

epithelial cells have keratin filaments, whereas endothelial cells have vimentin filaments. The lining of the buccal cavity is an example of unkeratinized, stratified epithelium, whereas the skin consists of dry, keratinized, stratified epithelium. Biomembranes may contain efflux transporters that move permeating drug molecules back to the membrane exterior and influx transporters that actively transport drug molecules through the membranes (Figure 2.43). *Mucosa* (mucus membrane) is an epithelial membrane containing mucosal cells that secret mucus, a gel-like fluid containing mainly water ($\sim 95\%$), mucins ($0.5-5\%$), inorganic salts ($\sim 1\%$), proteins ($0.5-1\%$), lipids, and mucopolysaccharides [23,24]. Mucins are large glycoproteins with molecular weight ranging from about 0.5 to 20 megadaltons (MDa). Some are membrane bound, but others are not. Mucin forms hydrogen bonds with surrounding water molecules, decreases water mobility, and forms an unstirred water layer (UWL) on the epithelial surface, the mucus layer. The mucus layer on the eye surface (i.e., the tear film) is about 5 μm thick, but the thickness of the GI mucus layer can be about 170 μm [24,25]. The UWL owes its existence to the cohesion properties of water, that is, the ability of water molecules to form hydrogen bonds with not only other water molecules but also hydrocarbons, proteins, glycoproteins (e.g., mucin), ions, and other membrane structures. UWLs such as mucus layers are hydrophilic barriers to absorption of lipophilic drugs [26].

2.10.2 Passive Transport Through Mucosa

Dissolved drug molecules are transported through the aqueous mucus layer, which is a UWL, via passive diffusion. The drug concentration gradient drives drug permeation through the UWL. Then, the drug molecules partition from the aqueous exterior into the lipophilic epithelium. Finally, the drug molecules are transported through the epithelium, probably mainly by passive diffusion via transcellular or paracellular route but also by influx transporters or carrier-mediated active transport. Efflux transporters actively transport drug molecules out of the cells and thus can hamper drug absorption through biomembranes (i.e., reduce drug bioavailability). Even drugs that are actively transported through membranes permeate the aqueous mucus layer via passive diffusion.

Figure 2.44 shows passive permeation of drug molecules through the mucosa, which is described as a simple bilayer membrane barrier, consisting of an aqueous mucus layer and a lipophilic epithelial layer. Bilayer membrane barrier to drug permeation can be described as additive resistances, the resistance (R_D) of an aqueous diffusion layer and the resistance (R_M) of a lipophilic membrane [27−29]. Assuming independent and additive resistances of the two layers, the total drug permeation resistance (R_T) of this simple membrane can be defined as:

$$R_T = R_D + R_M \tag{2.155}$$

Since the permeability constants (P) are the reciprocals of the resistances, the following equation is obtained assuming sink conditions (i.e., $C_S - C_D \approx C_S$ and $C_1 - C_2 \approx C_1$ in Figure 2.43):

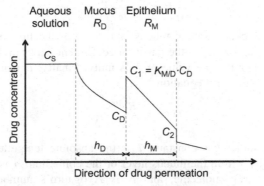

FIGURE 2.44   Passive permeation of dissolved drug molecules through mucosa.

$$J = P_T \cdot C_S = (R_D + R_M)^{-1} \cdot C_S = \left(\frac{1}{P_D} + \frac{1}{P_M}\right)^{-1} \cdot C_S \qquad (2.156)$$

where J is the drug flux from the aqueous mucus exterior through the membrane, P_T is the overall permeability coefficient, C_S is the concentration of dissolved drug in the aqueous mucus exterior, and P_D and P_M are the permeability coefficients in the mucus and within the membrane, respectively. Rearranging Eq. (2.156) gives:

$$J = \left(\frac{P_D \cdot P_M}{P_D + P_M}\right) \cdot C_S \qquad (2.157)$$

If permeation is much slower through the membrane itself than through the mucus (i.e., $P_D > P_M$), then:

$$J \approx \left(\frac{P_D \cdot P_M}{P_D}\right) \cdot C_S = P_M \cdot C_S \qquad (2.158)$$

In that case, the viscous mucus layer only has a negligible effect on drug permeation through the mucosa and can be ignored (i.e., $R_M > R_D$). This can, for example, be the case when relatively large and/or hydrophilic molecules permeate the mucosal epithelium. If, however, permeation through the epithelium is much faster than permeation through the mucus (i.e., $P_M > P_D$), then:

$$J \approx \left(\frac{P_D \cdot P_M}{P_M}\right) \cdot C_S = P_D \cdot C_S \qquad (2.159)$$

In this case, the mucus layer is the main barrier (i.e., $R_D > R_M$), and drug permeation through the mucosa becomes controlled by the aqueous diffusion layer. This can, for example, be the case when relatively small and lipophilic molecules permeate the mucosal epithelium. The relationship between the permeation coefficient (P) and the diffusion coefficient (D) is given by Eq. (2.160):

$$P = \frac{D \cdot K_{M/D}}{h} \qquad (2.160)$$

where h is the thickness of the mucus layer (h_D) or the lipophilic epithelial membrane (h_M), and $K_{M/D}$ is the partition coefficient between the membrane and the mucus. For P_D, the value of K is unity. Finally, D can be estimated from the Stokes−Einstein equation:

$$D \approx \frac{R \cdot T}{6\pi \cdot \eta \cdot r \cdot N} \qquad (2.161)$$

where R is the molar gas constant, T is the absolute temperature, η is the apparent viscosity within the mucus layer or the epithelium, r is the radius of the permeating drug molecule, and N is Avogadro's number. Thus, the diffusion constant within the mucus (D_D) will decrease with the increasing viscosity of the layer as well as with the increasing molecular weight of the drug. The presence of mucin in the mucus layer increases not only the thickness (h_D) of the UWL but also its viscosity (η), both of which will increase its resistance (R_D), consequently decreasing drug permeability though the UWL.

REFERENCES

[1] Kerc J, Opara J. A new amoxicillin/clavulanate therapeutic system: preparation, *in vitro* and pharmacokinetic evaluation. Int J Pharmaceut 2007;335:106–13.

[2] Wagner JG, Nelson E. Kinetic analysis of blood levels and urenary excretion in the absorptive phase after single dose of drug. J Pharm Sci 1964;53:1392–403.

[3] Burstein AH, Modica R, Hatton M, Forrest A, Gengo FR. Pharmacokinetics and pharmacodynamics of midazolam after intranasal administration. J Clin Pharmacol 1997;37:711–18.

[4] Bertucci C, Domenici E. Reversible and covalent binding of drugs to human serum albumin: methodological approaches and physiological relevance. Curr Med Chem 2002;9:1463–81.

[5] Vuignier K, Schappler J, Veuthey JL, Carrupt PA, Martel S. Drug–protein binding: a critical review of analytical tools. Anal Bioanal Chem 2010;398:53–66.

[6] Sweetman SC. Martindale. The complete dru reference. London: Pharmaceutical Press; 2002.

[7] Moffat AC, Osselton MD, Widdop B. Clarck's analysis of drugs and poisons. London: Pharmaceutical Press; 2004.

[8] Agwuh KN, MacGowan A. Pharmacokinetics and pharmacodynamics of the tetracyclines including glycylcyclines. J Antimicrob Chemother 2006;58:256–65.

[9] Fatemi MH, Ghorbannezhad Z. Supplimentary material to estimation of the volume of distribution of some pharmacologically important compounds from their structural descriptors. J Serb Chem Socv 2011;76:S7–10.

[10] Kurkov SV, Loftsson T. Cyclodextrins. Int J Pharmaceut 2013;453:167–80.

[11] Schwartz GJ, Haycock GB, Edelmann CM, Spitzer A. Simple estimate of glomerulalfiltration rate ib children derived from body length and plasma creatinine. Pediatrics 1976;58:259–63.

[12] Cockcroft DW, Gault MH. Prediction of creatinine clearance from serum creatinine. Nephron 1976;16:31–41.

[13] Kampmann J, Siersbaeknielse. K, Kristensen M, Hansen JM. Rapid evaluation of creatinine clearance. Acta Med Scand 1974;196:517–20.

[14] Levy G. Pharmacokinetics of salicylate elimination in man. J Pharm Sci 1965;54:958–67.

[15] Levy G, Tsuchiya T. Salicylate accumulation kinetics in man. N Engl J Med 1972;287:430–2.

[16] Dubovska D, Piotrovskij VK, Gajdos M, Krivosikova Z, Spustova V, Trnovec T. Pharmacokinetics of salicylic acid and its metabolites at low doses—a compartmental modeling. Methods Find Exp Clin Pharmacol 1995;17:67–77.

[17] Galinsky RE, Svensson CK. Basic pharmacokinetics and pharmacodynamics. In: Allen LV, editor. Remington, the science and practice of pharmacy. London: Pharmaceutical Press; 2013. p. 1073–93.

[18] Loftsson T. Drug stability for pharmaceutical scientists. Amsterdam: Academic Press; 2014.

[19] Borga O, Hoppel C, Odarcederlof I, Garle M. Plasma levels and rena excretion of phenytoin and its metabolites in patients with renal faliure. Clin Pharmacol Ther 1979;26:306−14.

[20] Fu SL, Molnar A, Bowron P, Lewis J, Wang HJ. Reduction of temazepam to diazepam and lorazepam to delorazepam during enzymatic hydrolysis. Anal Bioanal Chem 2011;400:153−64.

[21] Riss J, Cloyd J, Gates J, Collins S. Benzodiazepines in epilepsy: pharmacology and pharmacokinetics. Acta Neurol Scand 2008;118:69−86.

[22] Shou MG, Mei Q, Ettore MW, Dai RK, Baillie TA, Rushmore TH. Sigmoidal kinetic model for two co-operative substrate-binding sites in a cytochrome P450 3A4 active site: an example of the metabolism of diazepam and its derivatives. Biochem J 1999;340:845−53.

[23] Bansil R, Turner BS. Mucin structure, aggregation, physiological functions and biomedical applications. Curr Opin Colloid Interface Sci 2006;11:164−70.

[24] Lai SK, Wang YY, Wirtz D, Hanes J. Micro- and macrorheology of mucus. Adv Drug Deliver Rev 2009;61:86−100.

[25] Lai SK, Wang YY, Hanes J. Mucus-penetrating nanoparticles for drug and gene delivery to mucosal tissues. Adv Drug Deliver Rev 2009;61:158−71.

[26] Behrens I, Stenberg P, Artursson P, Kissel T. Transport of lipophilic drug molecules in a new mucus-secreting cell culture model based on HT29-MTX cells. Pharmaceut Res 2001;18:1138−45.

[27] Higuchi T. Physical chemical analysis of percutaneous absorption process from creams and ointments. J Soc Cosmet Chem 1960;11(2):85−97.

[28] Flynn GL, Carpenter OS, Yalkowsk SH. Total mathematical resolution of diffusion layer control of barrier flux. J Pharm Sci US 1972;61:312−14.

[29] Loftsson T, Brewster ME. Pharmaceutical applications of cyclodextrins: effects on drug permeation through biological membranes. J Pharm Pharmacol 2011;63:1119−35.

Chapter 3

Physicochemical Properties and Pharmacokinetics

Chapter Outline

The physicochemical properties of substances such as their aqueous solubility, ionization (pK_a), lipophilicity, number of hydrogen bond donors and acceptors, polar surface area, physical and chemical stability, and molecular shape and weight will affect their fate in our body, their pharmacokinetics, and our ability to convert biologically active compounds to therapeutically active drugs or use inactive compounds as pharmaceutical excipients [1]. A biologically active compound is said to have druglike properties if it has acceptable absorption, distribution, metabolism, and excretion (ADME)/Tox properties to survive through the completion of phase I trials in humans [2]. If a biologically active compound does not possess druglike properties, it will never be a marketed drug. A complete understanding of how physicochemical properties of active pharmaceutical ingredients (APIs) and pharmaceutical excipients affect their interactions with the human body is of essence to pharmaceutical formulators in their search for ever more effective drug delivery and improved therapeutic efficacy.

3.1 LIPINSKI'S RULE OF FIVE

Lipinski et al. [3] evaluated druglike properties of over 2,000 biologically active compounds (i.e., drugs and drug candidates) and came up with what is known as "Lipinski's rule of five." Due to its simplicity, this method is widely used by researchers to predict not only absorption of compounds from the gastrointestinal (GI) tract but also the overall druglike properties of

Essential Pharmacokinetics. DOI: http://dx.doi.org/10.1016/B978-0-12-801411-0.00003-2

biologically active compounds. The rule of five applies only to passive absorption and is based on the 90th percentile (i.e., 90% of the compounds that had sufficient oral absorption had physicochemical properties within the rule of five). Lipinski's rule of five (four prerequisites that are based on the number 5) states that poor absorption or permeation through the biomembrane is more likely when:

- there are more than 5 hydrogen-bond (H-bond) donors (expressed as the sum of all nitrogen—hydrogen and oxygen—hydrogen bonds),
- there are more than 10 H-bond acceptors (expressed as the sum of nitrogen and oxygen atoms),
- the molecular weight (M_w) is over 500, and
- the log $P_{octanol/water}$ is over 5.

However, compounds that are substrates for biologic transporters, for example, some antibiotics, are exceptions to the rule.

The physicochemical rationale for the Lipinski's rule of five is based on the fact that:

- In aqueous solutions, H-bonds are formed between water and dissolved molecules, and these H-bonds must be broken when the molecules partition from the aqueous exterior into the lipophilic membrane. The more H-bonds there are, the more difficult it becomes for the molecule to partition from the aqueous exterior into the membrane (i.e., $K_{M/D}$ in Eq. (2.160) will decrease with increasing number of H-bonds).
- M_w refers to the size of the molecule (i.e., the radius [r] of the permeating molecule). According to Eq. (2.161) the diffusion coefficient (D) decreases with increasing M_w (i.e., with increasing r). This decrease in D will decrease drug permeation through the biologic membranes Eq. (2.160). Furthermore, large molecules are generally less soluble than small molecules, and thus, the increase in M_w will generally decrease C_S in Eq. (2.157).
- Increase in the lipophilicity (e.g., increased log $P_{octanol/water}$) will decrease aqueous solubility and consequently decrease C_S in Eq. (2.157). Also, if the log is greater than 5, then the dissolved molecules will partition into the lipophilic membrane but will have less tendency to partition from the membrane on the receptor side into the aqueous internal layers.
- The efflux and influx transporters can reduce or enhance, respectively, drug absorption through the biologic membranes and thus impact drug absorption through the biologic membranes. The impact of the transporters is not predicted by Lipinski's rule of five.

Table 3.1 shows the number of H-bond donors and acceptors for six drugs and one excipient, as well as the M_w and calculated log $P_{octanol/water}$, and their oral bioavailability. Although the rule of five is based on oral drug absorption, it can be applied to predict drug permeation through the

TABLE 3.1 Rule of Five and Oral Bioavailability

	M_w (Da)	log $P_{o/w}$	H-bond donors	H-bond acceptors	Bioavailability after oral administration
Acetaminophen (Paracetamol), pK_a 9.5	151	0.5	2	3	90%
Chloramphenicol	323	1.1	3	7	70%
β-Cyclodextrin	1,135	−11	21	35	0.5–3%

(Continued)

TABLE 3.1 (Continued)

	M_w (Da)	log $P_{o/w}$	H-bond donors	H-bond acceptors	Bioavailability after oral administration
Doxorubicin, pK_a 8.2 and 10.2	544	1.3	7	12	5%
Prednisolone	360	1.6	3	5	80%
Streptomycin	582	−7.5	16	19	Low and variable
Tetracycline, pK_a 3.3, 7.7, 9.7	444	1.4	7	10	80%

Based on data from Refs. [4,5]

TABLE 3.2 The Limiting Rule of Five Values for Oral Bioavailability as well as for Transdermal, Ophthalmic, and Pulmonary Drug Delivery

Route of drug administration	M_w (Da)	log $P_{o/w}$	H-bond donors	H-bond acceptors
Oral drug delivery	500	5.0	5	10
Transdermal drug delivery	335	5.0	2	5
Topical drug delivery to the eye	500	4.2	3	8
Pulmonary drug delivery	500	3.4	4	10

Modified from Ref. [6]

biomembranes in general, although the effect of, for example, M_w and log P might vary for different membranes (Table 3.2). There are exceptions from Lipinski's rule of five, but it still gives important information on how the physicochemical properties of compounds direct their fate within the body, and this information leads to successful drug design and delivery. Close to half of the failures in drug development can be attributed to poor dissolution in aqueous media, poor membrane permeability through biomembranes, or both, which are the same physicochemical properties that have laid the foundation for the rule of five.

3.2 THE BIOPHARMACEUTICS CLASSIFICATION SYSTEM

In recognition of the fact that close to half of the failures in drug development can be traced to poor biopharmaceutical properties, namely, poor dissolution or poor permeability, Gordon Amidon introduced the Biopharmaceutics Classification System (BCS) [7]. According to the BCS, orally administered drugs are divided into four classes on the basis of their solubility and permeability characteristics [8]. Like the rule of five, the BCS is based on Eq. (2.156), on the values of P_T and C_S. In the BCS, a given drug substance is considered "highly soluble" (i.e., having high C_S) when the highest dose strength is soluble in 250 milliliters (ml) or less of water over a pH range 1−7.5 at 37°C and "highly permeable" (i.e., having high P_T) when the extent of oral absorption in humans is determined to be greater than 90% of an administered dose (in solution), based on mass-balance or related to an intravenous (IV) reference dose. Highly soluble, highly permeable drugs, that is, drugs possessing the ideal physicochemical properties, are termed *Class I compounds*. High-throughput discovery methods are, however, selective for difficult-to-formulate *Class II* and *Class IV compounds* (Table 3.3).

TABLE 3.3 The BCS is Based on the Aqueous Drug Solubility (C_S) Over the pH Range 1–7.5 and Permeability (P_T), and Potential Formulation Approaches

Class	C_S	P_T	Absorption rate control	Formulation approaches for oral administration
I	High	High	Gastric emptying	Can easily be formulated as tablets or capsules
II	Low	High	Dissolution	Particle size reduction (e.g., formation of microparticles or nanoparticles), solid dispersions, salt formation, addition of surfactants, self-emulsifying systems, liquid capsules, complexation
III	High	Low	Permeability	Addition of permeation enhancers, efflux inhibitors
IV	Low	Low	Dissolution and permeability	Combination of Class II and III approaches

Class I consists of water-soluble drugs (i.e., have high C_S) that are well absorbed from the GI tract (i.e., have high P_T) and, in general, have the preferred physicochemical properties for optimal oral bioavailability. For immediate-release dosage forms, the absorption rate will be controlled by the gastric emptying rate. However, to secure constant high bioavailability, the dissolution rate must be relatively fast, or over 85% of the labeled amount of drug substance dissolves within 30 min in less than 900 ml buffer solution. Drugs in Class I are frequently somewhat lipophilic with M_w less than 500 daltons (Da) and C_S 1 milligram per milliliter (mg/ml) or greater. Examples of Class I drugs are acetaminophen (paracetamol), piroxicam, and propranolol hydrochloride. Although the oral bioavailability of propranolol is somewhat low due to extensive first-pass metabolism (see Sections 1.1 and 2.6.2) the drug is still well absorbed from the GI tract and thus belongs to Class I.

Class II drugs, which are poorly soluble in water (C_S <0.1 mg/ml), when dissolved, are well absorbed from the GI tract (i.e., have high P_T). The dissolution rate in vivo is usually the rate-limiting step in drug absorption. Commonly, drugs in this class have variable absorption due to the numerous formulation effects and in vivo variables such as food intake, which can affect their dissolution. Different formulation techniques are applied to compensate for the insolubility of the drugs and the consequent slow dissolution rate (Table 3.3). Through these various formulation approaches, the formulator tries to "move" drugs from Class II to Class I without changing the intrinsic ability of the drug molecules to permeate the biomembranes.

TABLE 3.4 The Approximate Dose-to-Solubility Ratios (D:S) and Dissolution Requirements for Different Routes of Administration

Drug formulation	D:S	pH range	Dissolution requirements
Conventional oral tablets	≤250 ml	1−7.5	≥85% within 30 min
Fast-dissolving buccal tablets	≤2 ml	3−7.5	Close to 100% within 1 min
Vaginal tablets	<2 ml	3.5−4.9	−
Aqueous nasal spray	<0.5 ml	5−8.5	Solution
Aqueous eye drop solution	<0.05 ml	6.6−9	Solution

Examples of Class II drugs are carbamazepine, glibenclamide, ketoconazole, ketoprofen, nifedipine, and phenytoin.

Class III consists of water-soluble drugs (i.e., have high C_S), which do not readily permeate the biomembranes (i.e., have low P_T). For these drugs, the rate-limiting factor in drug absorption is their permeability. Including absorption-enhancing excipients (i.e., compounds that decrease the barrier properties of epithelia in the GI tract) in their formulation can enhance their bioavailability, but some Class III drugs are only marketed as parenteral solutions. Examples of Class III drugs available as tablets are acyclovir, atenolol, captopril, and ranitidine.

Class IV consists of poorly soluble drugs (i.e., have low C_S), which, when solubilized, do not readily penetrate the biomembranes (i.e., have low P_T). These drugs are usually very difficult to formulate for effective oral delivery. Examples of Class IV drugs are cyclosporin A and furosemide.

Although the BCS was originally developed for solid oral dosage forms, similar systems can be applied to other types of drug administration [9]. However, as Table 3.4 shows, solubility and permeability requirements differ for the different routes of administration. For example, the volume of the aqueous tear fluid is only about 7 microliters (μl), and after topical administration of aqueous eye drop solutions, most of the dissolved drug molecules are washed from the eye surface within a few minutes, resulting in drug bioavailability of less than 5%. The volume of an eye drop varies between 0.03 and 0.05 ml, and consequently, the drug dose must dissolve in less than 0.05 ml. A given drug that belongs to Class I when given orally can be in Class II when given in the form of eye drops or a nasal spray. For example, the solubility of diazepam in water (at room temperature) is 0.05 mg/ml. Diazepam and other benzodiazepines are primarily used as sedative−antianxiety drugs, but they do also possess antiepileptic properties. The normal dose of diazepam is 5 mg. The dose-to-solubility ratio (D:S) is 100, which is well below the upper limit of 250 for oral delivery. The oral bioavailability of diazepam has been reported to be close to 100%. When given orally, diazepam is a Class I drug. However, if diazepam is to be formulated as a nasal spray for treatment of seizures, the upper limit of the D:S is 0.3 ml, which makes it a Class II drug. Consequently, the formulation of an aqueous diazepam nasal spray that has good bioavailability can be quite difficult.

Regulatory authorities use the BCS in their evaluation of new drug products, For example, the US Food and Drug Administration (FDA) grants waivers of in vivo bioequivalence studies for immediate-release solid oral dosage forms containing Class I drugs [10].

3.3   THE BIOPHARMACEUTICS DRUG DISPOSITION CLASSIFICATION SYSTEM

The Biopharmaceutics Drug Disposition Classification System (BDDCS), which is based on drug solubility and metabolism, was introduced by Wu and Benet [11]. They observed that a great majority of BCS Class I and II drugs (i.e., drugs that possess high permeability) are primarily eliminated through metabolism (e.g., $Cl_H > Cl_R$ in Section 2.6.2), whereas the majority of BCS Class III and IV (i.e., drugs that possess low permeability) is primarily eliminated unchanged in urine (i.e., $Cl_H < Cl_R$). Furthermore, they observed that there is a strong correlation between the extent of metabolism and the intestinal permeability rate (i.e., drugs displaying high permeability according to the BCS also display extensive metabolism according to the BDDCS). Thus, although the definition of "highly soluble" (i.e., having high C_S) in the BDDCS is identical to that of BCS (i.e., drug is highly soluble when the highest dose strength is soluble in ≤ 250 ml water over a pH range $1-7.5$ at $37°C$), permeability can be replaced by the extent of drug metabolism (i.e., drug is extensively metabolized when $\geq 90\%$ of the drug dose is metabolized) (Table 3.5) [12]. Class I (high solubility, high permeability) drugs possess high solubility and high permeability. High concentrations of dissolved drug in the gut will result in saturation of both absorptive and efflux transporters, minimizing any transporter effects on absorption. Class II (low solubility, high permeability) drugs possess low solubility and the low concentrations of dissolve drug in the gut will prevent saturation of the efflux transporters. Consequently, efflux transporter effects predominate in the gut as well as in the liver. Class III (high solubility, low permeability) drugs possess high solubility and low permeability, which results in high concentrations of dissolved drug in the gut. However, absorptive transporters will be necessary to overcome low drug permeability, and thus, absorptive transporter effects will predominate. Class IV (low solubility, low permeability) drugs display both low solubility and low permeability, and thus, absorptive and efflux transporter effects can be important.

TABLE 3.5 The BDDCS is Based on the Aqueous Drug Solubility (C_S) Over the pH Range 1−7.5 and Metabolism

Class	C_S	Metabolism	Hepatic versus renal clearance	Oral dosing transporter effects
I	High	Extensive	$Cl_H > Cl_R$	Transporter effects minimal in gut and liver
II	Low	Extensive	$Cl_H > Cl_R$	Efflux transporter effects predominate in the gut, but both uptake and efflux transporters can affect liver metabolism
III	High	Poor	$Cl_H < Cl_R$	Absorptive transporter effects predominate
IV	Low	Poor	$Cl_H < Cl_R$	Absorptive and efflux transporter effects can be important

Finally, like the rule of five and the BCS, Wu and Benet's BDDCS, which is an extension of the BCS, has its limitations, and in every class, there are some exceptions. All three classification systems are somewhat oversimplified but can help us understand how the physicochemical properties of drugs affect their pharmacokinetics without drug-specific predictions. These tools can thus facilitate successful drug design and product formulation.

3.4   METABOLIZABILITY, SOFT DRUGS, AND PRODRUGS

The ADME properties of drugs and drug candidates can be altered through chemical modifications (Figure 3.1), that is, by introducing new chemical moieties in biologically active compounds (i.e., through prodrug design) or introduction of chemically labile bonds in biologically active compounds (i.e., through soft drug design). The aim of such chemical modifications of biologically active compounds is to affect their aqueous solubility (C_S), permeability (P_T), metabolizability, or all three. The result is new chemical entity with improved ADME/Tox properties.

Prodrugs are pharmacologically inactive (or weakly active) derivatives of active drugs that are obtained through chemical modifications of biologically active compounds (Table 3.6). They are designed to maximize the amount of active drug that reaches its site of action, through manipulation of the physicochemical, biopharmaceutical, or pharmacokinetic properties. The inactive prodrugs are converted into active drugs within the body through

Prodrug:

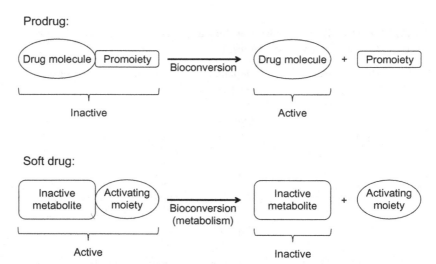

Soft drug:

FIGURE 3.1   The difference between pharmacologically inactive prodrug and pharmacologically active soft drug.

enzymatic or non-enzymatic reactions such as hydrolysis. For example, ampicillin is a hydrophilic zwitterionic drug that displays low solubility in the jejunum and small intestine (pH approximately 5−7) and, consequently, low bioavailability after oral administration (Table 3.7). Ampicillin pivaloyloxymethyl ester (pivampicillin) does not form zwitterion and displays relatively good solubility in water, although it is much more lipophilic than ampicillin. Consequently, the oral bioavailability of pivampicillin is almost twice that of ampicillin. Similarly, the valine ester of acyclovir (BCS Class III drug) increases the oral bioavailability of acyclovir and the 2-propanol ester of tafluprost acid increases its ocular bioavailability (Table 3.6). Some prodrugs are designed to prevent metabolism (e.g., docarpamine), whereas others allow their parenteral administration in aqueous solutions free of surfactants, and organic solvents (e.g., fosphenytoin).

Soft drugs are pharmacologically active derivatives of inactive and nontoxic compounds that can be hydrophilic metabolites of known drugs (Table 3.8). They are characterized by a predictable and controllable metabolism to nontoxic products after they have achieved their therapeutic role. Oxidative pathways are avoided as much as possible, since oxidation frequently leads to the formation of biologically active metabolites that can lead to adverse effects. Rather, chemically labile linkages such as ester linkages are introduced into biologically active compounds. This makes their metabolism much less dependent on saturable metabolic pathways. Thus, inactivation of soft drugs is not dose dependent (see Section 2.8) and much less dependent on liver and kidney (renal) functions (see Section 5.2).

TABLE 3.6 Examples of Drugs That Are Marketed as Prodrugs and Their Therapeutic Improvements

Drug (active)	Prodrug (inactive)	Improvement
Acyclovir	Valacyclovir	Results in about fivefold increase in oral bioavailability due to transporter-mediated absorption
Ampicillin	Pivampicillin	Converts poorly soluble but hydrophilic zwitterionic drug to somewhat lipophilic prodrug, resulting in enhanced oral bioavailability
Dopamine	Docarpamine	Prevents metabolism of dopamine in the intestine and liver, resulting in enhanced oral bioavailability
Lovastatin acid	Lovastatin	A natural product
Phenytoin	Fosphenytoin	Results in about 7,000-fold increase in aqueous solubility, allowing parenteral delivery of the drug in pure aqueous solution
Tafluprost acid	Tafluprost	Increases permeation from aqueous eye drops through the cornea, resulting in enhanced ocular bioavailability

TABLE 3.7 The Physiochemical Properties and Pharmacokinetic Parameters of Ampicillin (Broken Curves) and its Prodrug Pivampicillin (Solid Curves) in Humans

	Ampicillin	Pivampicillin
M_w (Da)	349	464
pK_a at 25°C	2.5 (–COOH), 7.3 (–NH$_2$)	7.0 (–NH$_2$)
Solubility in water at pH 5 and 25°C	0.2 mg/ml	2.4 mg/ml
pH 7 and 25°C	0.9 mg/ml	0.1 mg/ml
Calculated log $P_{octanol/water}$ at pH 5 and 25°C	1.0	2.2
pH 7 and 25°C	–1.6	3.7
Absolute bioavailability	47–49%	82–89%

Sketches showing the mean ampicillin plasma concentrations and the mean cumulative ampicillin urinary recovery after oral administration of 800 μmol of ampicillin or pivampicillin to healthy volunteers in a crossover study:

Data were collected from Refs. [4,13,14]

TABLE 3.8 Examples of Soft Drugs, Their Major Metabolite and Observed Therapeutic Improvements

Soft drug (active)	Metabolite (essentially inactive)	Improvement
Clevidipine	Clevidipine acid	This calcium channel blocker is rapidly metabolized by esterases in the blood and extravascular tissues and, thus, its half-life ($t_{1/2}$) is only a couple of minutes following parenteral administration (i.e., it is an ultra−short-acting calcium channel blocker)
Esmolol	Esmolol acid	This β_1-receptor antagonist is rapidly metabolized by esterases in blood to form a practically inactive metabolite, and thus, its $t_{1/2}$ is less than 10 min after parenteral administration
Loteprednol etabonate	Δ^1-Cortienic acid	This corticosteroid is susceptible to enzymatic and non-enzymatic hydrolysis, and this lowers its systemic exposure following topical administration to the eye
Remifentanil	Remifentanil acid	This ultra-fast short-acting synthetic opioid analgesic drug is rapidly metabolized by esterases in blood and tissues to form a practically inactive metabolite and, thus, its $t_{1/2}$ is considerably shorter ($t_{1/2}$ <15 min) than that of other opioids after parenteral administration

TABLE 3.9 The Physiochemical Properties and Pharmacokinetic Parameters in Humans of Fentanyl and its Soft Analog Remifentanil (Remifentanyl)

	Fentanyl	Remifentanil
Structure		
M_w (Da)	336	376
pK_a at 25°C	8.9	6.7
Solubility in water at pH 5 at 25°C	130 mg/ml	140 mg/ml
Calculated log $P_{octanol/water}$ at pH 7 at 25°C	2.2	1.7
Protein binding in plasma	80−85%	89−92%
$t_{1/2}$ of the elimination phase	About 4 h (dose dependent)	Less than 0.25 h (not dose dependent)

Data were collected from Refs. [4,13,15]

A typical soft drug is inactivated through simple hydrolysis to form a highly hydrophilic and biologically inactive metabolite that is then excreted from the body without further conversions (see Figure 2.39). For example, remifentanil has similar physical properties and pharmacologic activity as fentanyl, but remifentanil is metabolized by esterases that are widespread throughout the body to form hydrophilic metabolite, remifentanil acid, which is excreted unchanged in urine (Table 3.9). Remifentanil acid is 1,000−2,000 times less potent than remifentanil. The parent drug, fentanyl, is mainly metabolized by oxidases (e.g., cytochrome P450) in the liver, and thus, its excretion is highly dependent on the liver function.

3.5   PHARMACOKINETICS OF EXCIPIENTS

The mammillary model can also be used to describe the ADME of pharmaceutical excipients and other xenobiotics. Just like drugs, excipients follow one- or two-compartment models and display biologic half-lives (Table 3.10). We can also apply Lipinski's rule of five, the BCS, and the BDDCS to predict the biologic fate of novel pharmaceutical excipients and drug delivery systems. The absorption of pharmaceutical polymers from the GI tract will depend on their M_w. Many commonly used pharmaceutical polymers are highly

TABLE 3.10 Physicochemical Properties of Some Pharmaceutical Excipients and Their Pharmacokinetic Parameters in Healthy Human Volunteers; Logarithm of the Calculated Partition Coefficients Between 1-Octanol and Water at pH 7 and 25°C (log $P_{o/w}$), Solubility in Water at pH 7 and 25°C, and the Half-Life of the Elimination Phase ($t_{1/2}$)

Excipient	M_w (Da)	log $P_{o/w}$	Solubility (mg/ml)	Oral bioavailability (%)	$t_{1/2}$ (h)	Comments	Ref.
Aspartame	294	−2.0	44	Negligible	3.5	Metabolized rapidly in the gut wall	[16]
Dextran 1	1,000	<<0	Highly soluble	Very low	1.9	Mainly (80%) excreted unchanged in urine after parenteral administration	[17]
Dextran 60	60,000	<<<0	Highly soluble	Negligible	42	Mainly degraded in the liver to lower M_w product before being excreted from the body	[17,18]
HPβCD	1400	−11	>600	0.5–3	1.9	Mainly (>90%) excreted unchanged in urine after parenteral administration	[19]
Polyethylene glycol 3350 (PEG-3350)	3,000–3,700	−4	Highly soluble	Negligible[a]	5.8	Mainly (85%) excreted unchanged in feces after oral administration	[20,21]

(Continued)

TABLE 3.10 (Continued)

Excipient	M_w (Da)	log $P_{o/w}$	Solubility (mg/ml)	Oral bioavailability (%)	$t_{1/2}$ (h)	Comments	Ref.
Propylene glycol (PG)	76	−1.0	380	Studies indicate that PG is well absorbed from the GI tract	4.1[b]	About 45% is excreted unchanged in urine and about 55% metabolized in the liver	[22]
Saccharin sodium	205	−1.1	Highly soluble	>90	1.1	Mainly excreted unchanged in urine	[23]
Sucralose	398	−0.5	300	<15	13	Mainly (85%) excreted unchanged in feces after oral administration	[24]
SBEβCD	2163	<−10	>500	Negligible	1.8	Mainly (95%) excreted unchanged in urine after parenteral administration	[19,25]

Polymers such as dextran 1 and 60 and PEG-3350 are polydisperse (i.e., heterogenic mixture of different size molecules), where the M_w given is the weight average M_w, and the physiochemical and biologic properties reported are only observed values for a given product.
[a]Studies in rats have shown that jejunal permeation of PEG decreases rapidly with increasing M_w; from about 45% (M_w = 330 Da) to about 5% (M_w = 1,100 Da) [26].
[b]The half-life of PG has been reported to be significantly longer in children [27].

hydrophilic ($\log P$ well below 0), have a large number of H-bond acceptors and donors, and M_w well above 500 Da, and thus, they are not absorbed intact from the GI tract. In general, only small oligomers are absorbed, to some extent, from the GI tract after oral administration. Water-soluble starch derivatives that are commonly used as excipients in oral drug formulations frequently fall into BCS Class III (high solubility, low permeability). Normally, starches and other carbohydrates undergo enzymatic hydrolysis and bacterial digestion in the GI tract. Even small oligosaccharides such as cyclodextrins with M_w between 1,000 and 2,000 Da display very low oral bioavailability and undergo almost complete bacterial digestion in the GI tract [19]. Polymers such as dextrans, which consist of mixtures of closely related polysaccharides, mainly of the α-1,6-glucan type, are given in aqueous parenteral solutions as plasma expanders. The half-lives ($t_{1/2}$) of parenterally administered dextrans are governed by their M_w. Dextran 1 (average M_w about 1,000 Da) is readily excreted unchanged in humans by glomerular filtration with a $t_{1/2}$ of about 1.9 h, whereas dextran 60 (average M_w about 60,000 Da) is excreted much more slowly ($t_{1/2} \approx 42$ h) [18]. It has been shown that the M_w threshold for unrestricted glomerular filtration of dextran is about 15,000 Da and that dextrans with M_w above 50,000 Da are not eliminated unchanged via the renal route in any significant amount [28,29]. Similarly the elimination rate of other water-soluble polymers tends to decrease with increasing M_w and number of substituents [18]. Polyvinylpyrrolidone (PVP) is essentially not metabolized in the body, and consequently, only PVP with M_w below about 10,000 Da, which is readily eliminated by glomerular filtration, is used in parenteral solutions [30,31]. In general, only low M_w polymers (M_w below about 15,000 Da) are used as excipients in parenteral solutions.

Most pharmaceutical excipients came into use long before current regulatory requirements were installed, and thus, pharmacokinetic parameters for most excipients cannot be readily obtained from the literature. Cyclodextrins such as 2-hydroxypropyl-β-cyclodextrin (HPβCD) and sulfobutylether β-cyclodextrin (SBEβCD) are relatively new excipients that are mainly used as solubilizers of poorly soluble, lipophilic drugs in aqueous solutions and solid drug products. The pharmacokinetics of HPβCD and SBEβCD have been studied in humans, and it has been shown that they are mainly (i.e., 93−100%) excreted unchanged through glomerular filtration after parenteral administration [5,19,25,32,33]. Their plasma concentration−time profiles show a brief distribution phase, which is followed by an elimination phase (i.e., HPβCD and SBEβCD follow two-compartment model after IV injection). The $t_{1/2}$ of the elimination phase is 1.8−1.9 h, and their V_D is approximately 0.2 l/kg. Pharmacokinetic studies have shown that over 90% of parenterally administered HPβCD and SBEβCD will be eliminated from the body within approximately 6 h and over 99.9% within 24 h. Thus, no accumulation of CD will be observed in individuals with normal kidney function, even at high doses (Figure 3.2). However, cyclodextrin accumulation will be

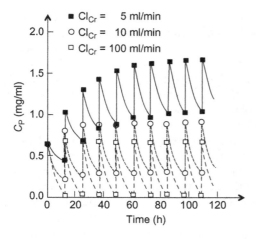

FIGURE 3.2 Predicted plasma cyclodextrin concentrations (C_P) after IV bolus administration of 10 g of cyclodextrin every 12 h ($D_0 = 10$ g, $\tau = 12$ h) in patients with normal kidney function ($Cl_{Cr} = 100$ ml/min) and severely decreased kidney function ($Cl_{Cr} = 10$ and 5 ml/min). Volume of distribution (V_D), 16 l; half-life ($t_{1/2}$) in patients with normal kidney function, 1.8 h; and fraction of cyclodextrin excreted unchanged in urine, 95% ($f_e = 0.95$) [19].

observed in patients with severe renal impairment, that is, individuals with creatinine clearance (Cl_{Cr}) below approximately 10 ml/min.

REFERENCES

[1]   Kerns EH, Di L. Drug-like properties: concepts, structure design and methods; from ADME to toxicity optimization. Amsterdam: Academic Press; 2008.

[2]   Lipinski CA. Drug-like properties and the causes of poor solubility and poor permeability. J Pharmacol Toxicol Methods 2000;44:235−49.

[3]   Lipinski CA, Lombardo F, Dominy BW, Feeney PJ. Experimental and computational approaches to estimate solubility and permeability in drug discovery and development settings. Adv Drug Deliver Rev 1997;23:3−25.

[4]   Moffat AC, Osselton MD, Widdop B. Clarck's analysis of drugs and poisons. London: Pharmaceutical Press; 2004.

[5]   Loftsson T, Brewster ME. Pharmaceutical applications of cyclodextrins: basic science and product development. J Pharm Pharmacol 2010;62:1607−21.

[6]   Choy YB, Prausnitz MR. The rule of five for non-oral routes of drug delivery: ophthalmic, inhalation and transdermal. Pharm Res 2011;28:943−8.

[7]   Amidon GL, Lennernas H, Shah VP, Crison JR. A theoretical basis for a biopharmaceutic drug classification: the correlation of in vitro drug product dissolution and *in vivo* bioavailability. Pharmaceut Res 1995;12:413−20.

[8]   FDA. The Biopharmaceutics Classification System (BCS) Guidance. <http://www.fda. gov/AboutFDA/CentersOffices/OfficeofMedicalProductsandTobacco/CDER/ucm128219. htm>; 2009.

[9]   Loftsson T. Cyclodextrins and the biopharmaceutics classification system of drugs. J Incl Phenom Macro 2002;44:63−7.

[10] Guidance for industry: Waiver of in vivo bioavailability and bioequivalence studies for immediate-release solid oral dosage forms based on a Biopharmaceutics Classification System. U.S. Food and Drug Administration (FDA), Center for Drug Evaluation and

Research (CDER). <http://www.gmp-compliance.org/guidemgr/files/3618FNL.PDF>; 2000.

[11] Wu CY, Benet LZ. Predicting drug disposition via application of BCS: Transport/absorption/elimination interplay and development of a Biopharmaceutics Drug Disposition Classification System. Pharmaceut Res 2005;22:11−23.

[12] Chen ML, Amidon GL, Benet LZ, Lennernas H, Yu LX. The BCS, BDDCS, and Regulatory Guidances. Pharmaceut Res 2011;28:1774−8.

[13] SciFinder. Chemical Abstracts Series. Washington, DC: American Chemical Society; 2014.

[14] Sjövall J, Magni L, Bergan T. Pharmacokinetics of bacampicillin compared with those of ampicillin, pivampicillin, and amoxycillin. Antimicrob Agents Chemother 1978;13:90−6.

[15] Beers R, Camporesi E. Remifentanil update. Clin Sci Utility, CNS Drugs 2004;18:1085−104.

[16] Puthrasingam S, Heybroek WN, Johnston A, Maskrey V, Swift CG, Turner P, et al. Aspartame pharmacokinetics—The effect of ageing. Age Ageing 1996;25:217−20.

[17] Schwarz JA, Koch W, Buhler V, Kaumeier S. Pharmacokinetics of low molecular (mono valent) dextran (DX-1) in volunteers. Int J Clin Pharmacol Ther 1981;19:358−67.

[18] Klotz U, Kroemer H. Clinical pharmacokinetic considerations in the use of plasma expanders. Clin Pharmacokinet 1987;12:123−35.

[19] Kurkov SV, Loftsson T. Cyclodextrins. Int J Pharmaceut 2013;453:167−80.

[20] Pelham RW, Nix LC, Chavira RE, Cleveland MV. P. Stetson, Clinical trial: single- and multiple-dose pharmacokinetics of polyethylene glycol (PEG-3350) in healthy young and elderly subjects. Aliment Pharmacol Ther 2008;28:256−65.

[21] Philipsen EK, Batsberg W, Christensen AB. Gastrointestinal permeability to polyethylene glycol: an evaluation of urinary recovery of an oral load of polyethylene glycol as a parameter of intestinal permeability in man. Eur J Clin Invest 1988;18:139−45.

[22] Yu DK, Elmquist WF, Sawchuk RJ. Pharmacokinetics of propylene glycol in humans during multiple dosing regimens. J Pharm Sci US 1985;74:876−9.

[23] Sweatman TW, Renwick AG, Burgess CD. The pharmacokinetics of saccharin in man. Xenobiotica 1981;11:531−40.

[24] Robersts A, Renwick AG, Sims J, Snodin DJ. Sucralose metabolism and pharmacokinetics in man. Food Chem Tox 2000;38:S31−41.

[25] Hafner V, Czock D, Burhenne J, Riedel KD, Bommer J, Mikus G, et al. Pharmacokinetics of sulfobutylether-beta-cyclodextrin and voriconazole in patients with end-stage renal failure during treatment with two hemodialysis systems and hemodiafiltration. Antimicrob Agents Chemother 2010;54:2596−602.

[26] Kim M. Absorption of polyethylene glycol oligomers (330−1122 Da) is greater in the jejunum that in the ileum of rats. J Nutr 1996;126:2172−8.

[27] De Cock RFW, Knibbe CAJ, Kulo A, de Hoon J, Verbesselt R, Danhof M, et al. Developmental pharmacokinetics of propylene glycol in preterm and term neonates. Br J Clin Pharmacol 2013;75:162−71.

[28] Arturson G, Granath K, Thoren I, Wallenius G. Renal excretion of low molecular weight dextran. Acta Chir Scand 1964;127:543−51.

[29] Arturson G, Wallenius G. The intravascular persistence of dextran of different molecular sizes in normal humans. Scand J Clin Lab Invest 1964;16:76−80.

[30] Schiller A, Reb G, Taugner R. Excretion and intrarenal distribution of low-molecular polyvinylpyrrolidone and inulin in rats. Arzneimittel-Forschung-Drug Res 1978;28:2064−70.

[31] Robinson BV, Sullivan FM, Borzelleca JF, Schwartz SL. A critical review of the kinetics and toxicology of polyvinylpyrrolidone (povidone). Chelsea, MI: Lewis Publishers; 1990.

[32] Zhou HH, Goldman M, Wu J, Woestenborghs R, Hassell AE, Lee P, et al. A pharmacokinetic study of intravenous itraconazole followed by oral administration of itraconazole capsules in patients with advanced human immunodeficiency virus infection. J Clin Pharmacol 1998;38:593−602.

[33] de Repentigny L, Ratelle J, Leclerc JM, Cornu G, Sokal EM, Jacqmin P, et al. Repeated-dose pharmacokinetics of an oral solution of itraconazole in infants and children. Antimicrob Agents Chemother 1998;42:404−8.

Chapter 4

Drug Pharmacokinetics After Alternative Routes of Administration

Chapter Outline

Previously, using the mammillary model, we described the drug pharmaco-kinetics of common pharmaceutical formulations such as tablets, capsules, and parenteral solutions. Identical mammillary models can also be used to describe drug pharmacokinetics after, for example, sublingual, nasal, rectal and vaginal delivery. Mammillary models can be constructed for other routes of administration such as topical drug delivery to the eye. Here, we provide a few examples of how the previously described models can be used in their present forms or with some minor modifications to describe alternative routes of drug delivery.

4.1 FENTANYL TRANSDERMAL PATCH

Fentanyl is a synthetic opioid analgesic that is 100-fold more potent than morphine. The physicochemical properties and pharmacokinetic parameters of the drug (Table 4.1) show that it does not violate Lipinski's rule of five with regard to transdermal drug delivery (see Table 3.2) and that the drug has, in fact, excellent transdermal bioavailability. Fentanyl permeates from a transdermal patch through the skin barrier via passive diffusion (see Section 2.10), according to Eq. (2.158) where the concentration gradient

Essential Pharmacokinetics. DOI: http://dx.doi.org/10.1016/B978-0-12-801411-0.00004-4

TABLE 4.1 Fentanyl, Structure, Physicochemical Properties, and Pharmacokinetic Parameters [2−4]

M_w (Da)	336
Solubility in water at pH 7 at 25°C	4 mg/ml
log $P_{octanol/water}$ at pH 7 and 25°C	3.68
H-bond acceptors	3
H-bond donors	0
$t_{1/2}$	1.5−7 h (dose dependent)
V_D	1−4 l/kg
Bioavailability:	
Oral	32% (first-pass metabolism)
Buccal	50%
Nasal	89%
Transdermal	92%

over the membrane barrier is the driving force (see Figure 2.44); no active transport is involved in transdermal drug delivery. Figure 4.1 shows the plasma fentanyl concentration in patients after transdermal drug delivery. The patch was removed from the skin after 24 hours (h), but the fentanyl plasma concentration was monitored for 2 days after the patch had been removed. The drug is released from the patch and permeates the skin barrier (i.e., stratum corneum) and then through the viable epidermis, where it is absorbed into the general blood circulation. The bioavailability of fentanyl from a transdermal patch has been determined to be 92%; in other words, on average, 92% of the drug released from the patch reaches the blood circulation after dermal application, and the other 8% of the drug is metabolized in the skin or degraded by the skin's bacterial flora [1]. The fentanyl plasma profile from a transdermal patch is very similar to the one shown in

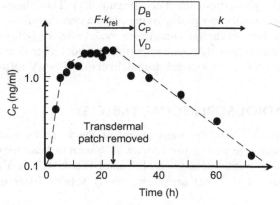

FIGURE 4.1   Semilog plot showing the mean fentanyl plasma concentration after administration of transdermal fentanyl patch for 24 h to eight patients. The drug released (k_{rel}) from the patch is 100 micrograms per hour ($\mu g/h$), but some fraction of the drug does not reach the general blood circulation, and consequently, the bioavailability (F) is less than unity. *Sketch based on data from Ref. [1].*

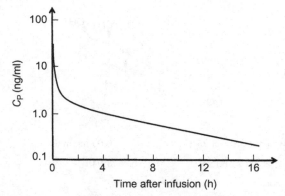

FIGURE 4.2   Sketch of a semilog plot showing the fentanyl plasma concentration after slow (5 min) IV bolus administration of fentanyl ($D_0 = 0.75$ mg) to patients. *Based on data from Ref. [1].*

Figure 2.7, a profile of a drug that follows the one-compartment open model after administration by intravenous (IV) infusion (see Figure 2.4). Plasma concentration (C_P) increases and then levels off into a plateau ($C_P = C_{SS}$; see Figure 2.16) at about 12 h, when the rate of drug delivery is equal to the rate of drug elimination from the body. After the patch has been removed, the C_P declines according to first-order kinetics (i.e., fentanyl is eliminated from the body according to the one-compartment open model). Although fentanyl follows the two-compartment open model after IV bolus injection [2], the plasma profile appears to follow the one-compartment model after transdermal delivery. The relatively short distribution phase, which is clearly seen in the plasma profile after IV injection (Figure 4.2), disappears into the slow drug absorption phase from the patch (Figure 4.1). This phenomenon is not uncommon. Frequently, drugs displaying plasma concentration–time profiles that follow the two- or three-compartment model after IV bolus injection display profiles that follow the one-compartment model after slow delivery, for example, after oral or transdermal drug delivery or slow IV infusion.

4.2 ESTRADIOL SUBLINGUAL TABLETS

Estradiol (17β-estradiol), the most potent of the naturally occurring estrogens, is frequently given to postmenopausal women to treat, for example, hot flashes and to prevent osteoporosis. Estradiol (Table 4.2) is a potent (daily IV dose about 0.1–0.2 mg) lipophilic, poorly soluble (0.09 milligram per

TABLE 4.2 17β-Estradiol, Structure, Physicochemical Properties, and Pharmacokinetic Parameters [5,6]

M_w (Da)	272
Solubility in water at pH 7 at 25°C	0.09 mg/ml
log $P_{octanol/water}$ at pH 7 and 25°C	3.94
H-bond acceptors	2
H-bond donors	2
Normal 17β-estradiol plasma levels:	
Premenopausal women	110–1500 pmol/L (30–400 pg/ml)
Postmenopausal women	<220 pmol/L (<60 pg/ml)
Terminal $t_{1/2}$ of exogenous 17β-estradiol	3.5 h
Bioavailability:	
Oral	5% (extensive first-pass metabolism)
Sublingual (buccal)	25%
Nasal	80%
Transdermal	≤100%

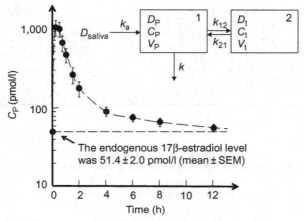

FIGURE 4.3 Semilog plot showing the mean estradiol plasma concentration after administration of 100 µg estradiol sublingual tablet to five postmenopausal women. The drug follows the two-compartment model with first-order drug absorption (see Figure 2.22 and Eq. (2.79)). *Sketch based on data from Ref. [6].*

milliliter [mg/ml]) drug of low molecular weight. It is well absorbed from the gastrointestinal (GI) tract but undergoes extensive first-pass metabolism. Estradiol is a Biopharmaceutics Classification System (BCS) Class I drug, which relatively easily permeates biologic membranes such as the nasal mucosa and skin. Most frequently, estradiol is administered in the form of transdermal patches, but it has been administered in the form of nasal sprays and fast-dissolving sublingual tablets. The plasma profile obtained after sublingual administration of estradiol (Figure 4.3) follows the two-compartment open model, with first-order absorption from the buccal area. The observed estradiol plasma concentrations are both due to endogenous estradiol and the exogenous estradiol from the sublingual tablets. The pharmacokinetic parameters are estimated in Example 4.1.

EXAMPLE 4.1 Sublingual Administration and Two-Compartment Model

The pharmacokinetic parameters of estradiol in sublingual tablets were determined during their development [6]. Each tablet contained 100 microgram (µg) of estradiol in a water-soluble complex with 2-hydroxypropyl-β-cyclodextrin. Five postmenopausal women (50–65 years old; 52–77 kg) received one sublingual tablet each, blood samples were drawn for up to 12 h from drug administration, and the plasma estradiol concentration was determined. The table shows the mean values (± standard error of the mean [SEM]) in the five women. Their basic estradiol plasma level (i.e., their level of endogenous estradiol) was determined to be 51.4 ± 2.0 picomoles per liter (pmol/L). Calculate the pharmacokinetic parameters of Eq. (2.79).

Time (h)	C_P (pmol/l) Total	Exogenous[a]	Time (h)	C_P (pmol/l) Total	Exogenous[a]
0.25	1083.6 ± 243.1	1032.2	2.0	180.6 ± 38.5	129.2
0.50	1032.2 ± 217.2	980.8	4.0	92.8 ± 12.4	41.4
0.75	734.8 ± 154.8	683.4	6.0	77.2 ± 8.0	25.8
1.00	485.0 ± 99.9	433.6	8.0	68.2 ± 8.4	16.8
1.50	270.2 ± 64.1	218.8	12.0	57.3 ± 6.3	5.9

[a]$C_{P\,Exo}$, $C_{P\,Tot} - C_{P\,Endo} = C_{P\,Tot} - 51.4 ± 2.0$ (pmol/l).

Answer

We apply the feathering technique to obtain the parameters, as shown in Example 2.8:

Eq. (2.78): $C_P = Ae^{-a \cdot t} + Be^{-b \cdot t} - Ce^{-k_a \cdot t}$

Time (h)	C_P (pmol/L)	$\ln C_P$	$(C_P - C'_P)$ (pmol/L)	$\ln(C_P - C'_P)$	$C''_P - (C_P - C'_P)$ (pmol/L)	$\ln(C''_P - (C_P - C'_P))$
0.25	1032.2	6.939	926.9	6.832	463.1	6.140
0.50	980.8	6.888	881.9	6.782		
0.75	683.4	6.459	590.4	6.381		
1.00	433.6	6.072	346.0	5.846		
1.50	218.8	5.388	141.3	4.951		
2.0	129.2	4.861	60.5	4.103		
4.0	41.4	3.723				
6.0	25.8	3.250				
8.0	16.8	2.821				
12.0	5.9	1.775				

$C''_P - (C_P - C'_P) = C \cdot e^{-k_a \cdot t}$ or

$\ln(C''_P - (C_P - C'_P)) = \ln C - k_a \cdot t$

$C'_P = B \cdot e^{-b \cdot t}$ or

$\ln C'_P = \ln B - b \cdot t$

$C''_P = (C_P - C'_P) = A \cdot e^{-a \cdot t}$ or

$\ln C''_P = \ln(C_P - C'_P) = \ln A - a \cdot t$

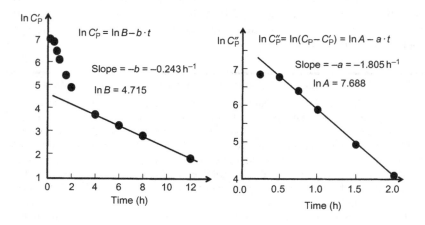

$\ln C'_P = \ln B - b \cdot t$

Slope $= -b = -0.243\,h^{-1}$

$\ln B = 4.715$

$\ln C''_P = \ln(C_P - C'_P) = \ln A - a \cdot t$

Slope $= -a = -1.805\,h^{-1}$

$\ln A = 7.688$

$A = e^{7.688} = 2{,}183 \text{ pmol/l}; \quad B = e^{4.715} = 111.6 \text{ pmol/l}; \quad C = ?$ (insufficient data)
$a = 1.81 \text{ h}^{-1}; \quad b = 0.24 \text{ h}^{-1}; \quad k_a = ?$ (insufficient data).

The calculated half-lives ($t_{1/2}$) of the elimination and the distribution phase are 2.8 h and 0.38 h, respectively. Only one point is observed in the absorption phase, and thus C and k_a in Eq. (2.79) cannot be determined. However, the plots indicate that maximum plasma concentration (C_{max}) is obtained at about 15 min ($t_{max} \approx$ 15 min).

4.3 DIAZEPAM SUPPOSITORIES

Diazepam is a benzodiazepine anxiolytic drug, which is used to treat anxiety and seizures such as status epilepticus. It is a BCS Class I drug and is generally well absorbed from the GI tract and when given intranasally or rectally (Table 4.3). However, the bioavailability of diazepam depends on the

TABLE 4.3 Diazepam, Structure, Physicochemical Properties, and Pharmacokinetic Parameters [4,7,8]

M_w (Da)	285
Solubility in water at pH 7 and 25°C	0.05 mg/ml
log $P_{octanol/water}$ at pH 7 and 25°C	2.80
pK_a	3.40
H-bond acceptors	3
H-bond donors	0
Terminal $t_{1/2}$	43 ± 13 h
Bioavailability:	
Oral	90–100%
Rectal	90%
Nasal	75–95%

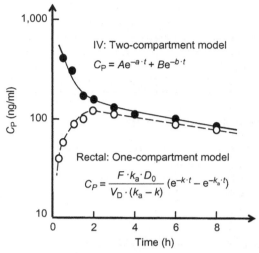

FIGURE 4.4 Semilog plot showing the mean diazepam plasma concentration after administration of 10 mg diazepam via bolus IV injection (●) or rectally in a suppository containing 10 mg diazepam (○). *Sketch based on data from Ref. [9].*

composition of its formulation. For example, diazepam is more rapidly absorbed and displays higher rectal bioavailability when it is administered in solution or hydrogel than when it is administered in a solid suppository. Diazepam is distributed according to the two-compartment model when given via IV bolus injection with a distribution phase (t from 0 to about 2 h) and an elimination phase (from t about 2 h) displaying a terminal $t_{1/2}$ (i.e., half-life of the drug in the elimination phase after absorption and distribution) of between 1 and 2 days (Figure 4.4). When given rectally in suppositories, diazepam is relatively slowly absorbed into the systemic blood circulation, and then the C_P versus time profile (Figure 4.4) is best described using the one-compartment open model with first-order drug absorption (see Section 2.4.2). After rectal administration, the distribution phase disappears into the absorption phase.

4.4   MIDAZOLAM NASAL SPRAY

Midazolam, like diazepam, is a benzodiazepine anxiolytic drug, which is used to treat anxiety, but its $t_{1/2}$ is much shorter or only about 2 h compared with 43 h for diazepam. Midazolam is mainly used to produce preoperative sedation. It is a BCS Class I drug and is generally well absorbed from the GI tract. However, midazolam displays low oral bioavailability due to first-pass metabolism, but the drug has shown reasonably good bioavailability after

TABLE 4.4 Midazolam, Structure, Physicochemical Properties, and Pharmacokinetic Parameters [4,10,11]

M_W (Da)	326
Solubility in water at pH 7 at 25°C	0.01 mg/ml
log $P_{octanol/water}$ at pH 7 and 25°C	3.76
pK_a	6.03
H-bond acceptors	3
H-bond donors	0
Terminal $t_{\frac{1}{2}}$	2 h
Bioavailability:	
Oral	36% (first-pass metabolism)
Rectal	52%
Nasal	73%

intranasal delivery (Table 4.4). However, the nasal bioavailability of midazolam will depend on the composition of its formulation. The nasal bioavailability of midazolam was determined to be 39% when midazolam parenteral solution was administered nasally (see Example 2.9) but 73% when it was administered in an aqueous cyclodextrin solution. The difference in bioavailability is due to the differences in dissolved midazolam in the two formulations, 5 mg/ml in the parenteral solution versus 17 mg/ml in the cyclodextrin-based nasal solution (Figure 4.5) [10]. Thus, relatively large amounts of the parenteral solution have to be sprayed into the nose to induce sedation and anxiolysis. Subsequently, midazolam is only partly absorbed from the nasal cavity and partly from the GI tract after it is swallowed.

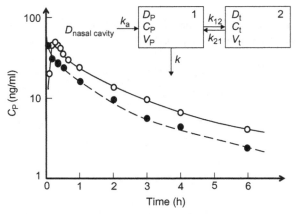

FIGURE 4.5 Semilog plot showing the mean midazolam plasma concentration in six healthy volunteers after administration of 2 mg fixed dose midazolam via bolus IV injection (●) or intranasally 0.06 milligram per kilogram (mg/kg) (○). *Sketch based on data from Ref. [10].*

4.5 PULMONARY DELIVERY (INHALATION) AND SUBCUTANEOUS INJECTION OF INSULIN

The human insulin is a small globular protein (M_w 5,808 daltons [Da]) that consists of 51 amino acid residues in two polypeptide chains, chain A (21 residues) and B (31 residues), which are linked by two disulfide bonds in addition to one disulfide loop in chain A (Table 4.5). It is slightly soluble in water but practically insoluble in organic solvents such as ethanol. After IV bolus injection, regular insulin, which is an endogenous compound, gives an immediate peak and C_P−time profile that is best fitted to the two-compartment open model with an initial $t_{1/2}$ of about 10 minutes (min) and terminal $t_{1/2}$ of a couple of hours. After subcutaneous (SC) insulin injection, the drug is absorbed into the blood circulation, giving C_{max} after about 90 min (Figure 4.6). The C_P−time profile after pulmonary insulin administration (inhalation) shows a C_{max} at about 20 min. The relative bioavailability of pulmonary versus SC administration is less than about 25% [12]. Insulin violates all of Lipinski's rule of five and thus only displays limited permeation through the biologic membranes (Table 4.5).

4.6 TOPICAL DELIVERY OF DEXAMETHASONE TO THE EYE

The most common ophthalmic drug formulation is aqueous eye drops. Typically, less than 5% of the topically applied drug dose is absorbed from aqueous eye drops into the eye. Most of the dose is washed with the tear fluid through the lacrimal ducts and eventually into the nasal cavity, where is absorbed into the systemic blood circulation. Dexamethasone is a potent,

TABLE 4.5 Human Insulin, Physicochemical Properties and Pharmacokinetic Parameters [13,14]

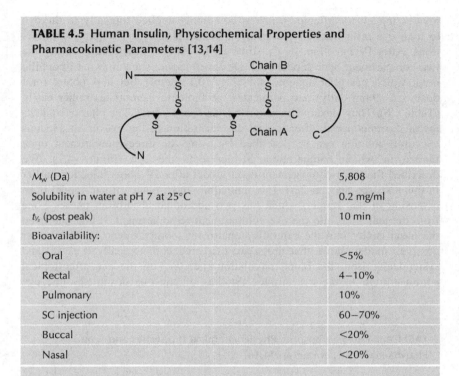

M_W (Da)	5,808
Solubility in water at pH 7 at 25°C	0.2 mg/ml
$t_{1/2}$ (post peak)	10 min
Bioavailability:	
Oral	<5%
Rectal	4–10%
Pulmonary	10%
SC injection	60–70%
Buccal	<20%
Nasal	<20%

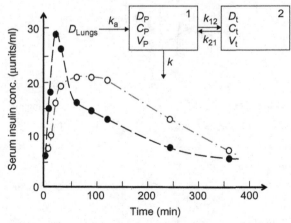

FIGURE 4.6 Semilog plot showing the serum insulin concentration in 18–24 healthy volunteers after administration of insulin by SC injection (○, dose 10.4 units) and by inhalation (●, dose 76.0 units). *Sketch based on data from Refs. [12,15]. One unit of human insulin is equivalent to 0.0347 mg.*

long-acting glucocorticoid, which is commonly applied topically to the eye to treat eye inflammation caused by, for example, injury, surgery, or infections. After IV injection, its C_P–time profile is best described by using the two-compartment open model [16]. Dexamethasone is a somewhat lipophilic drug, which has poor aqueous solubility (0.1 mg/ml), but it is potent (oral dose: 0.5–9 mg daily) and permeates the biologic membranes rather easily (Table 4.6). Thus, dexamethasone is a BCS Class I drug. The pharmacokinetics of dexamethasone after topical administration to the eye in an aqueous eye drop solution can be described by using the three-compartment open model, in which compartment 3 represents the eye (Figure 4.7). We described the three-compartment open model after IV bolus injection earlier in this text (see Section 2.3). The ophthalmic three-compartment model is an extension of that model, which has two additional absorption phases—one from the tear fluid into the eye compartment (compartment 3) and one from the nasal cavity into the central compartment (compartment 1). This rather complex model shows that drugs are delivered both topically (i.e., k_a') and systemically from the blood circulation (i.e., k_{13}) to the eye after topical administration to the eye surface. Studies of aqueous dexamethasone eye

TABLE 4.6 Dexamethasone, Physicochemical Properties and Some Pharmacokinetic Parameters [4,16]

M_w (Da)	392
Solubility in water at pH 7 at 25°C	0.11 mg/ml
log $P_{octanol/water}$ at pH 7 and 25°C	1.8
H-bond acceptors	5
H-bond donors	3
$t_{1/2}$	4.6 ± 1.2 h
V_D	1 l/kg
Oral bioavailability:	80%
Plasma protein binding	70%

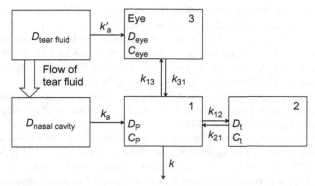

FIGURE 4.7 Mammillary three-compartment open model of topical delivery of dexamethasone in aqueous eye drop solution. The drug is delivered to the eye surface where a small fraction (<5%) of the drug is absorbed into the eye (i.e., compartment 3). Most of the drug (>90%) is washed away with the tear fluid into the nasal cavity, where it is absorbed into the systemic blood circulation (i.e., the central compartment or compartment 1) and distributed into the tissue compartment (i.e., compartment 2). D_P, amount of drug in central compartment; C_P, plasma concentration of the drug; D_t, amount of drug in tissue compartment; C_t, hypothetical drug tissue concentration; D_{eye}, amount of drug in the eye (compartment 3); C_{eye}, hypothetical eye concentration of the drug; k'_a, the first-order rate constant for drug absorption from the tear fluid into the eye; k_a, the first-order rate constant for drug absorption from the nasal cavity into compartment 1; k, overall first-order elimination rate constant; k_{12}, transfer rate constant from compartment 1 to compartment 2; k_{21}, transfer rate constant from compartment 2 to compartment 1; k_{13}, transfer rate constant from compartment 1 to compartment 3; k_{31}, transfer rate constant from compartment 3 to compartment 1.

drop solutions in rabbits have shown that although over 90% of dexamethasone in the anterior part of the eye (e.g., aqueous humor) is delivered via the topical route, a somewhat smaller fraction (or about 50%) of dexamethasone found in the posterior segment (e.g., vitreous humor and retina) is delivered via this route, and the rest reaches the eye via the systemic blood circulation [17]. However, although the weight of a normal laboratory rabbit is only about one-twentieth of that of a human, the rabbit eye is not much smaller than the human eye. Thus, pharmacokinetic studies of eye drops in rabbits may lead to overestimation of systemic drug delivery to the human eye.

REFERENCES

[1] Varvel JR, Shafer SL, Hwang SS, Coen PA, Stanski DR. Absorption characteristics of transdermally administered fentanyl. Anesthesiology 1989;70:928−34.
[2] Lötsch J, Walter C, Parnham MJ, Oertel BG, Geisslinger G. Pharmacokinetics of non-intravenous formulations of fentanyl. Clin Pharmacokinet 2013;52:23−36.
[3] Streisand JB, Varvel JR, Stanski DR, Lemaire L, Ashburn MA, Hague BI, et al. Absorption and bioavailability of oral transmucosal Fentanyl citrate. Anesthesiology 1991;75:223−9.
[4] SciFinder, in, Chemical Abstracts Series, American Chemical Society, 2014.

[5] Loftsson T, Hreinsdottir D. Determination of aqueous solubility by heating and equilibration: a technical note. Aaps PharmSciTech 2006;7: [article number 4].

[6] Loftsson T, Gudmundsson JA, Arnadottir RO, Fridriksdottir H. Sublingual delivery of 17 beta-estradiol from cyclodextrin containing tablets. Pharmazie 2003;58:358−9.

[7] Ivaturi V, Kriel R, Brundage R, Loewen G, Mansbach H, Cloyd J. Bioavailability of Intranasal vs. Rectal Diazepam. Epilepsy Res 2013;103:254−61.

[8] Cloyd JC, Lalonde RL, Beniak TE, Novack GD. A single-blind, crossover comparison of the pharmacokinetics and cognitive effects of a new diazepam rectal gel with intravenous diazepam. Epilepsia 1998;39:520−6.

[9] Dhillon S, Oxley J, Richens A. Bioavailability of diazepam after intravenous, oral and rectal administration in adult epileptic patients. Br J Clin Pharmacol 1982;13:427−32.

[10] Loftsson T, Guomundsdottir H, Sigurjonsdottir JF, Sigurosson HH, Sigfusson SD, Masson M, et al. Cyclodextrin solubilization of benzodiazepines: formulation of midazolam nasal spray. Int J Pharm 2001;212:29−40.

[11] Clausen TG, Wolff J, Hansen PB, Larsen F, Rasmussen SN, Dixon JS, et al. Pharmacokinetics of midazolam and α-hydroxy-midazolam following rectal and intravenous administration. Br J Clin Pharmacol 1988;25:457−63.

[12] Patton JS, Platz RM, Baldock SC. Methods and compositions for pulmonary delivery of insulin. In: E.P.A.N. 2036541, editor. 2009.

[13] Owens DR. New horizons—Alternative routes for insulin therapy. Nat Rev Drug Discov 2002;1:529−40.

[14] Kumar A, Pathak K, Bali V. Ultra-adaptable nanovesicular systems: a carrier for systemic delivery of therapeutic agents. Drug Discov Today 2012;17:1233−41.

[15] Man CD, Rizza RA, Cobelli C. Meal simulation model of the glucose-insulin system. IEEE Trans Biomed Eng 2007;54:1740−9.

[16] Czock D, Keller F, Rasche FM, Haussler U. Pharmacokinetics and pharmacodynamics of systemically administered glucocorticoids. Clin Pharmacokinet 2005;44:61−98.

[17] Sigurdsson HH, Konraosdottir F, Loftsson T, Stefansson E. Topical and systemic absorption in delivery of dexamethasone to the anterior and posterior segments of the eye. Acta Ophthalmol Scand 2007;85:598−602.

Chapter 5

Pharmacologic Response and Drug Dosage Adjustments

Chapter Outline

In general, drugs are administered on the basis of their average pharmacokinetic parameters in normal patient populations. Frequently, this is acceptable, achieves the desired therapeutic effect, and does not cause any adverse effects. Many drugs such as most over-the-counter (OTC) drugs and some antibiotics (e.g., penicillins and tetracyclines) have a wide therapeutic window (therapeutic index [TI] or therapeutic range; see Sections 1.1 and 2.7) and are easily maintained within the window, whereas others such as digoxin, aminoglycosides, antiarrhythmic drugs, and anticonvulsants (e.g., phenytoin) have a narrow therapeutic window and are more difficult to administer. In some cases, a strict individualization of the drug dose may be required. Figure 5.1 shows calculated phenytoin C_P–time curves in three different individuals, with phenytoin metabolized at an average rate ($t_{1/2} = 21$ h), fast ($t_{1/2} = 10$ h), and slowly ($t_{1/2} = 42$ h), when one 100 mg tablet is given three times a day ($D_0 = 100$ mg, $t = 8$ h). After the drug has been administered for about 3 days, the C_P reaches the minimum effective concentration (MEC) in the patient with $t_{1/2} = 21$ h, and the therapeutic effect is observed. The C_P never goes above minimum toxic concentration (MTC), and thus toxic side effects are never observed in the patient. In the fast-metabolizing patient, C_P never goes above the MEC and consequently, the therapeutic effect is never observed in this patient. The dosage (D_0) has to be increased (e.g., $D_0 = 250$ mg, $\tau = 8$) to elevate C_P above the MEC. In the slow-metabolizing patient, the therapeutic effect is observed after the drug has been administered for about 2 days, but after 4 days, toxic side effects start to be observed. Thus, the dose has to be lowered in the slow metabolizer (e.g., $D_0 = 50$ mg, $\tau = 8$).

Essential Pharmacokinetics. DOI: http://dx.doi.org/10.1016/B978-0-12-801411-0.00005-6

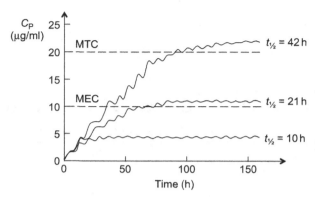

FIGURE 5.1 Sketch showing the drug concentration–time curves after administration of phe-nytoin that has a half-life ($t_{1/2}$) of about 22 h, with a range of 7–42, in three different individuals. The drug dose (D_0) is 100 mg given every 8 h ($\tau = 8$ h).

5.1 THERAPEUTIC DRUG MONITORING

Pharmacokinetic parameters of drugs such as rate constants and volumes of distributions may vary with patient's age, gender, weight, clinical status, nutritional status, genetic variability (slow or fast metabolism), and co-administration of two or more drugs (drug interactions). Therapeutic drug monitoring (TDM) is a branch of clinical pharmacokinetics that involves determination of plasma drug concentrations and subsequent change of the drug dosage to maintain plasma concentrations within a targeted therapeutic window or, in other words, to tailoring a dose regimen to an individual patient. TDM may be needed when during drug therapy, the patient does not show a proper therapeutic response or displays toxic drug reactions that can be related to low or high drug plasma concentrations (C_P). TDM is also used to monitor for a patient's compliance, that is, to check if the patient follows the prescribed drug regimen. In the beginning, patients receive standard dosage regimens based on information obtained from, for example, clinical handbooks and the drug manufacturer. If the patient displays inadequate therapeutic response or toxic symptoms, blood samples are collected and the drug plasma concentration determined. This is followed by pharmacokinetic evaluation of the data and dosage adjustment.

EXAMPLE 5.1 Dosage Adjustment of Theophylline

The following information on the pharmacokinetic parameters of theophylline was found in a clinical handbook:

Total body clearance (Cl_T) = 3 l/h
Biologic half-life ($t_{1/2}$) = 8 h
Volume of distribution (V_D) = 0.5 l/kg
Therapeutic index (TI) = 10–20 µg/ml

Minimum toxic concentration (MTC) = 20 µg/ml

Dosage regimen for a 70 kg patient: 250 mg four times a day (D_0 = 250 mg, τ = 6 h)

Oral bioavailability (F) is close to 100% ($F \approx 1.0$).

A patient (70 kg) received theophylline (two immediate-release tablets, each containing 125 mg theophylline) according to this dosage regimen but did not respond to therapy. The average plasma concentration (C_{av}^{∞}) was determined and shown to be only 6.0 µg/ml. Adjust the drug dosage regimen for this patient. Propose an alternative drug formulation on the basis of your results.

Answer

We use Eq. (2.135) to calculate new dosage regimen, assuming that the low is due to faster metabolism and keeping F, V_D, and τ unchanged:

$$C_{av}^{\infty} = \frac{F \cdot D_0}{V_D \cdot k \cdot \tau} = \frac{F \cdot D_0 \cdot t_{1/2}}{V_D \cdot \ln 2 \cdot \tau}$$

In this patient: 6.0 mg/l = $(1.0 \cdot 250 \cdot t_{1/2}/35\, l \cdot \ln 2 \cdot 6\,h)$ or $t_{1/2}$ = 3.5 h but $t_{1/2}$ is 8 h in a "normal" patient. If all pharmacokinetic parameters are identical except $t_{1/2}$, then the following equation can be derived from Eq. (2.135):

$$D_0' \cdot t_{1/2}' = D_0 \cdot t_{1/2} \text{ or } D_0' = D_0 \cdot \frac{t_{1/2}}{t_{1/2}'} = 250 \cdot \frac{8.0\,h}{3.5\,h} = 571\,mg$$

The new dosage regimen is then 571 mg four times a day (D_0 = 571 mg, τ = 6 h). Although this regimen will give C_{av}^{∞} within 10–20 µg/ml, the maximum (C_{max}) and minimum (C_{min}) theophylline plasma concentrations will be above and below the TI. If we give somewhat smaller dose such as four 125 mg tablets for times a day (D_0 = 500 mg, τ = 6 h), the following C_{max}^{∞} and C_{min}^{∞} can be estimated using Eqs. (2.120) and (2.121) for IV bolus administration (see Sections 2.7.1 and 2.7.3):

$$C_{max}^{\infty} = \frac{D_0}{V_D} \cdot \left(\frac{1}{1 - e^{-k \cdot \tau}}\right) = \frac{D_0}{V_D} \cdot \left(\frac{1}{1 - e^{-\left(\ln 2/t_{1/2}\right) \cdot \tau}}\right)$$

$$C_{max}^{\infty} = \frac{500\,mg}{35\,l} \cdot \left(\frac{1}{1 - e^{-(\ln 2/3.5) \cdot 6}}\right) = 20.55\,mg/l = 20.55\,\mu g/ml$$

$$C_{min}^{\infty} = \frac{D_0}{V_D} \cdot \left(\frac{1}{1 - e^{-k \cdot \tau}}\right) \cdot e^{-k \cdot \tau} = \frac{D_0}{V_D} \cdot \left(\frac{1}{1 - e^{-\left(\ln 2/t_{1/2}\right) \cdot \tau}}\right) \cdot e^{-\left(\ln 2/t_{1/2}\right) \cdot \tau}$$

$$= C_{max}^{\infty} \cdot e^{-\left(\ln 2/t_{1/2}\right) \cdot \tau}$$

$$C_{min}^{\infty} = C_{max}^{\infty} \cdot e^{-\left(\ln 2/t_{1/2}\right) \cdot \tau} = 20.55\,\mu g/ml \cdot e^{-(\ln 2/3.5) \cdot 6} = 6.26\,\mu g/ml$$

Since C_P goes below the MEC and above the MTC, this dosage regimen is not acceptable. To keep C_P within the TI, we would have to give smaller doses of theophylline more frequently, for example, 2½ tablet (D_0 = 312.5 mg) every 3 h (τ = 3 h): C_{av}^{∞} = 15.0 µg/ml, C_{max}^{∞} = 19.9 µg/ml and C_{min}^{∞} = 11.0 µg/ml. Such regimen is not practical, and thus theophylline is administered in sustained-release tablets (see Section 2.7.3) to avoid C_P fluctuations. Common dosage regimen for sustained-release theophylline tablets is $200-300$ mg every 12 h ($D_0 = 200-300$ mg, $\tau = 12$ h). This regimen for sustained-release theophylline tablets keeps C_P well within the TI.

5.2 DOSAGE ADJUSTMENTS

Kidneys and liver are the most important organs for drug elimination from the body. Any changes in their function will affect the drug $t_{1/2}$, as well as other pharmacokinetic parameters, and dosage adjustments will be required to maintain C_P within the therapeutic concentration range. Decreased kidney function (i.e., renal failure) can be due to, for example, infection, diabetes, or nephrotoxic drugs. It is mainly observed as a decreased glomerular filtration rate (GFR, see Section 2.6.2) or, in other words, decreased or absence of urine production. Dosage adjustments are also performed during dialysis (hemodialysis) when the blood of patients with acute kidney failure is treated in a dialysis machine (i.e., artificial kidney). Decreased liver function (i.e., hepatic failure) can be caused by, for example, excessive alcohol consumption, drug overdose (e.g., acetaminophen [paracetamol] overdose), and viral infection (e.g., hepatitis). Furthermore, both kidney and liver functions are affected by aging. The GFR declines with increasing age as does the metabolic rate; thus, older people are, in general, given smaller drug doses compared with young adults or middle-aged persons. Likewise, infants, especially newborns, do not have fully developed enzyme systems and generally require relatively small drug doses. Furthermore, newborns show only $30-40\%$ renal activity, according to body weight, in comparison with adults.

The equations used to adjust drug dosage are based on keeping the same C_{av}^{∞} in normal and affected persons, as described by Eq. (2.135), assuming that drug bioavailability is not affected (i.e., $F = F'$):

$$C_{av}^{\infty} = \frac{F \cdot D_0}{V_D \cdot k \cdot \tau} = \frac{F \cdot D_0}{Cl_T \cdot \tau} = \frac{F \cdot D_0 \cdot t_{1/2}}{V_D \cdot \ln 2 \cdot \tau} \text{ or } C_{av}^{\infty} = \frac{F \cdot D_0}{Cl_T \cdot \tau} = \frac{F' \cdot D_0'}{Cl_T' \cdot \tau'}$$

where the unmarked parameters (F, D_0, Cl_T, and τ) refer to the normal person but the marked parameters (F', D_0', Cl_T', and τ') refer to the patient with decreased kidney function, decreased liver function, or both.

$$\frac{D_0}{Cl_T \cdot \tau} = \frac{D_0'}{Cl_T' \cdot \tau'} \tag{5.1}$$

If $\tau = \tau'$:

$$\frac{D_0}{Cl_T} = \frac{D_0'}{Cl_T'} \tag{5.2}$$

$$D_0' = D_0 \cdot \frac{Cl_T'}{Cl_T} \tag{5.3}$$

If both τ and V_D do not change (e.g., during parenteral administration when D_0 can be changed by adjusting the injection volume):

$$D_0' = D_0 \cdot \frac{t_{\frac{1}{2}}}{t_{\frac{1}{2}}'} = D_0 \cdot \frac{k'}{k} \qquad (5.4)$$

If C_{av}^{∞} is kept constant by changing τ but both D_0 and V_D do not change (e.g., during oral administration of tablets or capsules where D_0 is fixed):

$$\tau' = \tau \cdot \frac{k}{k'} = \tau \cdot \frac{t_{\frac{1}{2}}'}{t_{\frac{1}{2}}} \qquad (5.5)$$

Or when both τ and D_0 are changed to maintain C_{av}^{∞} constant:

$$\frac{D_0'}{\tau'} = \frac{Cl_T'}{Cl_T} \cdot \frac{D_0}{\tau} = \frac{k'}{k} \cdot \frac{D_0}{\tau} \qquad (5.6)$$

Following are few examples of dosage adjustments.

EXAMPLE 5.2 Dosage Adjustment of Vancomycin

According to clinical handbooks, $t_{\frac{1}{2}}$ of vancomycin is 5.6 ± 1.8 h, and about 90% of the drug is excreted unchanged in urine. Vancomycin (7−10 mg/kg) is given by intravenous (IV) bolus injection every 8 h ($\tau = 8$ h) to patients with normal renal function. Determine the vancomycin dose for a 80 kg patient under the following conditions: (a) when $Cl_{cr} = 20$ ml/min and (b) under complete renal shutdown ($Cl_{cr} = 0$ ml/min).

Vancomycin is a glycopeptide antibiotic (M_w 1,449 Da) with 33 H-bond acceptors and 21 H-bond donors and thus displays negligible oral absorption.

Answer
In normal patients: $k = \ln 2/t_{\frac{1}{2}} = 0.693/5.6$ h $= 0.124$ h^{-1}. According to Eq. (2.71) $k = k_e + k_{nr}$. We also know that k_e is 90% of k ($k_e = 0.90 \cdot k$) and k_{nr} is 10% of k ($k_{nr} = 0.10$ k). In a patient with a normal kidney function $Cl_{cr} \approx 100$ ml/min (see Section 2.6.2), $k_e = 0.90 \cdot 0.124$ h$^{-1} = 0.112$ h^{-1} and $k_{nr} = 0.1 \cdot 0.124$ h$^{-1} = 0.012$ h^{-1}.

Also, let us assume that a normal 80 kg patient is given 650 mg every 8 h ($D_0 = 650$ mg, $\tau = 8$ h).

a. $k_{nr}' = k_{nr}$ and

$$k' = k_e' + k_{nr}' = \frac{20}{100} \cdot k_e + k_{nr} = 0.20 \cdot 0.112 \text{ h}^{-1} + 0.012 \text{ h}^{-1} = 0.0344 \text{ h}^{-1}$$

Then we apply Eq. (5.4) to calculate new dose where $\tau = \tau'$:

$$D_0' = D_0 \cdot \frac{k'}{k} = 650 \text{ mg} \cdot \frac{0.0344}{0.124} = 180 \text{ mg every 8 h}$$

b. When $Cl_{cr} = 0$ ml/min then $k_e = 0$ and $k' = k_{nr} = 0.012$ h^{-1}:

$$D_0' = D_0 \cdot \frac{k'}{k} = 650 \text{ mg} \cdot \frac{0.012}{0.124} \approx 65 \text{ mg every 8 h}$$

EXAMPLE 5.3 Dosage Adjustment of Gentamycin

The serum creatinine concentration in a woman (35 years, 80 kg) was determined to be 2.0 mg/100 ml. The woman is to receive gentamicin. Patients with normal renal function receive 2 mg/kg loading dose and then 1.5 mg/kg every 8 h. Gentamicin is an aminoglycoside antibiotic and is almost exclusively excreted unchanged via glomerular filtration. Calculate the dosage regimen for the woman.

Answer
Decreased renal function will not affect the loading dose:

$$D_L = 2 \text{ mg/kg} \cdot 80 \text{ kg} = 160 \text{ mg}$$

Then, the maintenance dose is determined on the basis of Cl_{cr} (e.g., Eq. (2.101)):

$$Cl_{cr} = \frac{[140 - \text{age(years)}] \cdot \text{body weight(kg)}}{72 \cdot C_{cr} \text{ (mg/100 ml)}} = \frac{[140 - 35] \cdot 80}{72 \cdot 2.0} = 58 \text{ ml/min}$$

For females, the value obtained is multiplied by 0.90, and thus Cl_{cr} for the woman is 52 ml/min. For gentamicin, $k_{NR} \approx 0$ and Cl_T is directly proportional to Cl_{cr}. Thus, we can use Eq. (5.3) to determine the maintenance dose for the woman:

$$D_0' = D_0 \cdot \frac{Cl_T'}{Cl_T} = D_0 \cdot \frac{Cl_{cr}'}{Cl_{cr}} = 1.5 \text{ mg/kg} \cdot \frac{52}{100} = 0.78 \text{ mg/kg or } 0.78 \cdot 80 = 62 \text{ mg}$$

The woman should be given 62 mg gentamicin every 8 h ($D_0 = 62$ mg, $\tau = 8$ h).

EXAMPLE 5.4 Dosage Adjustment in Dialysis

A patient receiving anticancer therapy is on dialysis. The flow rate (Q) of blood through the artificial kidney is 180 ml/min, corresponding to a plasma flow of 100 ml/min. The drug plasma concentration was determined to be 10 ng/ml in plasma entering the artificial kidney machine (C_a) and 2.5 ng/ml in plasma flowing from the machine (C_v). The clearance (Cl_T) of the drug is 10 ml/min when the patient is not undergoing dialysis. How should drug dosage be changed when the patient is connected to the artificial kidney machine?

Answer
Clearance is defined as the rate of elimination divided by the plasma concentration (Eq. (2.95)). For the artificial kidney machine (Cl_D), it is:

$$Cl_D = \frac{\text{rate of elimination}}{\text{plasma concentration}} = \frac{Q \cdot (C_a - C_v)}{C_P} = \frac{100 \text{ l/min} \cdot (10 - 2.5) \text{ ng/ml}}{10 \text{ ng/ml}}$$

$$= 75 \text{ ml/min}$$

$$Cl_T = 10 \text{ ml/min and } Cl_T' = Cl_T + Cl_D = 10 \text{ ml/min} + 75 \text{ ml/min} = 85 \text{ ml/min}$$

$$D'_0 = D_0 \cdot \frac{Cl'_T}{Cl_T} = D_0 \cdot \frac{85}{10} = 8.5 \cdot D_0$$

The drug dose needs to be increased 8.5-fold during the time the patient is on the kidney machine.

5.3 PHARMACODYNAMICS

Pharmacodynamics is the science that describes the relationship between the drug concentration at the receptor and the drug effect, also called *pharmacologic response* (see Figure 1.1). The drug receptor can, for example, be a well-defined place within the body (e.g., protein molecule inside or on the surface of a cell), or it can be on or within microorganisms or parasites that are located within the body or on its surface. At the receptor site, the drug (D) binds (i.e., forms a complex) with the receptor (R). True receptors are receptors for endogenous substances such as hormones, neurotransmitters, cytokines, and growth factors. In addition to these true receptors, drug receptors can be, for example, enzymes, transporters, structural proteins, and ion channels, which do not act as receptors for endogenous compounds. The relationship between the drug concentration at the receptor site and the drug effect is hyperbolic and looks like the Langmuir adsorption isotherm (Figure 5.2A). At high drug concentrations, the drug effect approaches a maximum value where 100% drug response is obtained. At this concentration, virtually all receptors have formed a drug–receptor complex (D–R). A sigmoidal relationship is obtained when the effect is plotted against the logarithm of the drug concentration (Figure 5.2B). The drug concentration that produces 50% of the maximum effect (EC_{50}) is determined from the linear section of the semilog plot.

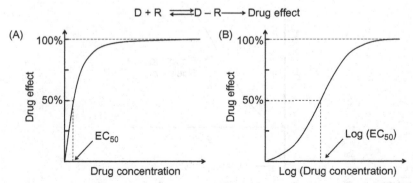

FIGURE 5.2 Schematic illustrations showing the drug concentration–response relationship on a linear scale (A) and as a semilog plot (B).

The drug effect shown in Figure 5.2A is thought to be proportional to the fraction of receptors occupied by drug molecules:

$$\text{Drug effect } (\%) = \frac{[D-R]}{[R]+[D-R]} \cdot 100 \tag{5.7}$$

where $[R]$ is the concentration of unoccupied receptor and $[D-R]$ is the receptor concentration that is occupied by drug molecules. Figure 5.2B shows that there is a linear relationship between the total drug concentration $(\log[D]_T)$ and the effect between approximately 20% and 80% drug effect. In this region the drug effect is proportional to the plasma drug concentration (C_P) as shown in Figure 5.3:

$$E = m \cdot \log[D]_T + e = m \cdot \log C_P + e \tag{5.8}$$

Rearranging Eq. (5.8) gives:

$$\log C_P = \frac{E - e}{m} \tag{5.9}$$

Equation (2.6) shows the first-order drug elimination from the body after IV bolus injection in the one-compartment open model. Replacing the natural logarithm in Eq. (2.6) with the common logarithm gives:

$$\log C_P = \log C_P^0 - \frac{k \cdot t}{2.303} \tag{5.10}$$

where C_P^0 is the drug plasma concentration at $t = 0$. Combining Eqs. (5.9) and (5.10) gives Eq. (5.11), where E_0 is the drug effect at $\log C_P^0$:

$$\frac{E - e}{m} = \frac{E_0 - e}{m} - \frac{k \cdot t}{2.303} \tag{5.11}$$

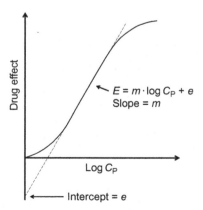

FIGURE 5.3   Typical log C_P versus drug effect (pharmacologic response) curve.

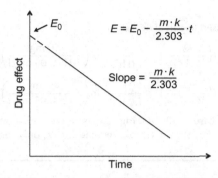

FIGURE 5.4 Drug effect (E) versus time (t) profile showing the linear decline with time. Note that the slope is the product of m, which is the proportionality constant between effect and drug concentration, and the first-order rate constant (k) for drug elimination divided by 2.303, which is the conversion factor between natural logarithm and common logarithm.

$$E = E_0 - \frac{m \cdot k \cdot t}{2.303} \tag{5.12}$$

Thus, in theory, the first-order drug elimination constant can be calculated by monitoring the changes in the drug effect (i.e., the pharmacologic response) with time (Figure 5.4).

Duration of drug action (t_{eff}) is the difference between the time for the drug concentration to fall back to the MEC (or C_{eff}) and the onset time (see Figure 1.3). For a drug that follows the one-compartment model after IV bolus injection, the following equation for duration can be derived from Eq. (2.6):

$$t_{eff} = \frac{\ln C_P^0 - \ln C_{eff}}{k} = \frac{\ln(D_0/V_D) - \ln C_{eff}}{k} = \frac{1}{k} \cdot \ln\left(\frac{D_0}{V_D \cdot C_{eff}}\right) \tag{5.13}$$

Since both V_D and C_{eff} are constants $-\ln(V_D \cdot C_{eff})$ is just a new constant:

$$t_{eff} = \frac{1}{k} \cdot \ln D_0 + \text{constant} \tag{5.14}$$

EXAMPLE 5.5 Drug Dose and Duration

A drug has a minimum effective plasma concentration (C_{eff}) of 0.05 µg/ml, its first-order elimination constant (k) is $1.0\,h^{-1}$, and its V_D is 20 l. The drug is administered by IV bolus injection, and its pharmacokinetics follows the one-compartment open model. Calculate t_{eff} when 50 and 500 mg are administered. Why does the 10-fold increase in D_0 not result in a 10-fold increase in t_{eff}?

Answer

Equation (5.13) is used to calculate t_{eff}:

$$t_{eff} = \frac{1}{k} \cdot \ln\left(\frac{D_0}{V_D \cdot C_{eff}}\right) = \frac{1}{1.0\,h^{-1}} \cdot \ln\left(\frac{50\,mg}{20\,l \cdot 0.05\,mg/l}\right) = 3.9\,h$$

$$t_{eff} = \frac{1}{k} \cdot \ln\left(\frac{D_0}{V_D \cdot C_{eff}}\right) = \frac{1}{1.0\,h^{-1}} \cdot \ln\left(\frac{500\,mg}{20\,l \cdot 0.05\,mg/l}\right) = 6.2\,h$$

When D_0 is increased 50–500 mg t_{eff} is increased from 3.9 to 6.2 h. Because $E \propto \log C_P$ (Eq. 5.9), a 10-fold increase in D_0 only results in a 1.6-fold increase in t_{eff}.

Agonists are drugs (e.g., dopamine) that bind and activate receptors (i.e., produce stimulus). *Antagonists* are drugs (e.g., propranolol) that bind to receptors without activating them and thus can prevent the binding of agonists that activate the receptors. Two different drugs that bind to the same receptor may have different *affinity* for the receptor. Drug A in Figure 5.5 has greater affinity for the receptor (i.e., is more potent) than drug B, but both drugs have the same efficacy (i.e., give the same maximum effect). Drug C has lower potency as well as lower efficacy than drugs A and B. Drugs that are competitive antagonists (e.g., atropine and propranolol) bind reversibly with receptors. They compete with agonists (e.g., endogenous substances such as neurotransmitters or exogenous compounds such as drugs) for a binding to the same receptor and thus decrease their potency; the curves are shifted to the right with increasing antagonist concentration (Figure 5.6A). Competitive antagonists decrease the apparent potency of an agonist (i.e., EC_{50} increases) but do not affect the agonist's efficacy. Drugs that are noncompetitive antagonists (e.g., phenoxybenzamine) bind irreversibly (e.g., through covalent binding) with receptors and thus effectively decrease the number of available receptors in the system (EC_{50} does not

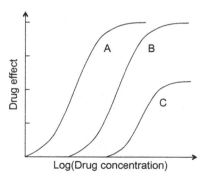

FIGURE 5.5 Drug A is more potent than drug B, but both drugs show the same efficacy. Drug C shows both lower potency and lower efficacy compared with drugs A and B.

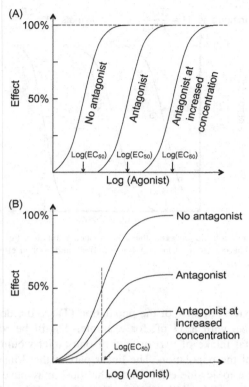

FIGURE 5.6 Sketches showing competitive inhibition (A), where both the agonist an antagonist bind reversibly to the receptor, and non-competitive inhibition by increasing concentration of an antagonist (B), where the antagonist binds irreversibly to the receptor.

change). Decreasing the number of available receptors will reduce the efficacy (Figure 5.6B). Unlike with competitive antagonists, the effect of noncompetitive antagonists cannot be reversed by increasing the concentration of the agonist. Some noncompetitive antagonists bind to an allosteric site on the receptor, that is, a separate binding site from the agonist, thus preventing receptor activation upon agonist binding or even prevent agonist binding.

Drugs often bind to more than one type of receptor and, consequently, produce more than one type of biologic effect. Besides the desired drug effect (pharmacologic response), various types of adverse, even lethal, effects can be observed. In Section 1.1, we defined the therapeutic concentration range of a drug as the concentration range from the MEC to the MTC. In animal studies, the TI is the lethal dose of a drug for 50% of the animal population (LD_{50}) divided by the minimum effective dose for 50% of the population (ED_{50}). In humans, TI is usually defined as the ratio of the dose

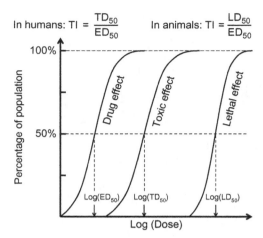

In humans: $TI = \dfrac{TD_{50}}{ED_{50}}$ In animals: $TI = \dfrac{LD_{50}}{ED_{50}}$

FIGURE 5.7 The relationship between the dose−response relationships for producing the desired drug effect (pharmacologic response), a toxic effect, and a lethal effect (see Section 1.1 and Eqs. (1.3) and (1.4)).

that produces toxicity in 50% of the population (TD_{50}) divided by ED_{50} (see Figure 1.4). Drugs with a TI of, for example, 2, will be relatively unsafe because accidental intake of two instead of one tablet would result in toxic effects in 50% of the population. The linear part of the drug dose−response relationships for a toxic side effect and lethal dose may have slopes that are different from those of the desired drug effect (Figure 5.7).

Although most drugs act by binding to specific receptors within the body, a few act by much simpler mechanisms that relate to their physicochemical properties. For example, antacids such as aluminum hydroxide, magnesium hydroxide, and calcium carbonate are bases that act by directly neutralizing gastric acidity, and chronic lead poisoning is treated with parenteral administration of an ethylenediaminetetraacetic acid (EDTA) complexing agent in the form of aqueous edetate disodium calcium (Ca−EDTA complex) solution. Calcium in the complex is readily replaced by lead (Pb^{2+}) to form the Pb−EDTA complex, which is excreted in urine.

Chapter 6

The Effect of Food and Excipients on Drug Pharmacokinetics

Chapter Outline

Food products, herbal medicines, dietary supplements, pharmaceutical excipients, co-administered drugs, and other chemicals can alter drug pharmacokinetics and consequently the therapeutic efficiency of a drug treatment. Their effect can be chemical (e.g., accelerated drug degradation in the gastrointestinal [GI] tract) or physical (e.g., enhanced or decreased aqueous solubility), or they can affect enzyme activity and active transport through inhibition or activation. Pharmacokinetic studies can give important information on how various xenobiotics affect the therapeutic efficacy of drugs. Such studies can give pharmaceutical formulators important information on excipient selection, that is, which one to use and which one to avoid. Furthermore, pharmacokinetic studies can tell patients which food products and herbal medicines they can safely consume during a given drug treatment and which they should avoid and also give information about drug–drug interactions. A few examples are discussed below.

Food, especially fatty food, is known to enhance the oral bioavailability of some poorly water-soluble, lipophilic drugs such as carbamazepine and griseofulvin by increasing their dissolution rate in the GI tract. Food may enhance the oral bioavailability of drugs by reducing their fist-pass metabolism (e.g., propafenone [Figure 6.1], metoprolol, and propranolol) or by delaying gastric emptying (e.g., phenytoin and spironolactone). Food can also delay drug absorption from the GI tract. For example, high-fiber foods are known to reduce the oral bioavailability of digoxin through the formation of digoxin–fiber complexes. Digoxin tablets are best taken on an empty stomach, especially if the patient is on a high-fiber diet. Tetracycline antibiotics form hydrophilic complexes (chelates) with various metal ions such

Essential Pharmacokinetics. DOI: http://dx.doi.org/10.1016/B978-0-12-801411-0.00006-8
131

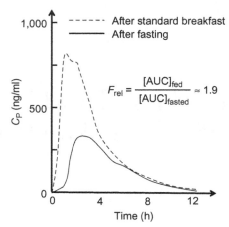

$$F_{rel} = \frac{[AUC]_{fed}}{[AUC]_{fasted}} \approx 1.9$$

FIGURE 6.1 Plot showing the propafenone plasma concentration in one healthy volunteer after 300 mg propafenone taken on an empty stomach and after receiving breakfast. *Sketch based on Ref. [1].*

as iron (Fe^{2+}), zinc (Zn^{2+}), magnesium (Mg^{2+}), and calcium (Ca^{2+}). These metal complexes, which consist of one metal ion and two tetracycline molecules, increase the apparent molecular weight of the parent drug, tetracycline, from 444 daltons (Da) to well over 900 Da, as well as the number of hydrogen bond acceptors and donors. Consequently, the bioavailability of tetracycline is significantly reduced upon formation of metal complexes (Figure 6.2). Dairy products, antacids, and iron supplements should not be consumed during tetracycline treatment. Cyclodextrins are enabling pharmaceutical excipients that enhance aqueous solubility of many lipophilic drugs [3]. Glibenclamide is a hypoglycemic agent that is practically insoluble in water, and consequently, drug dissolution in the GI tract is the rate-limiting step in its absorption (i.e., that glibenclamide is a Biopharmaceutics Classification System [BCS] Class II drug). In a canine study, the absolute bioavailability (F) of the pure drug (i.e., $F = [AUC]_{oral}/[AUC]_{IV}$) was determined to be 14.7%, whereas that of the complex was 90.5% [4]. Administering the drug as a water-soluble drug—cyclodextrin complex resulted in over a sixfold increase in the oral bioavailability of glibenclamide (Figure 6.3).

It is known that certain chemicals found in food can act as enzyme inhibitors and thus alter drug pharmacokinetics. For example, grapefruit juice can increase the plasma concentration of numerous drugs, especially those that undergo extensive first-pass metabolism. Chemicals (e.g., naringin and bergamottin) in grapefruit juice inhibit the CYP3A4 drug-metabolizing enzyme in the small intestine. This increases the drug plasma concentration (i.e., the area under the curve [AUC]) and maximum plasma concentration (C_{max}) [5].

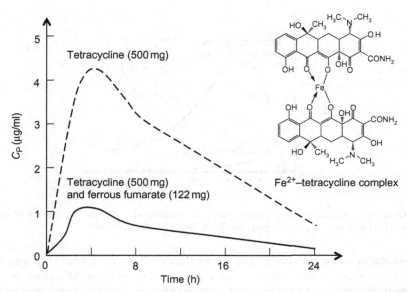

FIGURE 6.2 Plot showing the tetracycline plasma concentration in healthy volunteers after 500 mg tetracycline, taken either alone or with 122 mg of ferrous fumarate. Co-administration of a water-soluble iron salt results in about 80% reduction in the tetracycline bioavailability. *Sketch based on Ref. [2].*

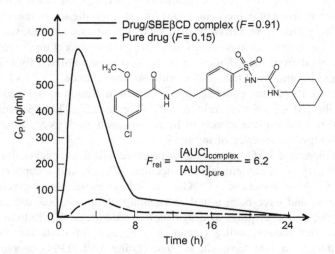

FIGURE 6.3 Plot showing the glibenclamide plasma concentration in dogs after administration of capsules containing 3.0 mg glibenclamide, either pure or in a complex with sulfobutylether β-cyclodextrin (SBEβCD). *F* is the absolute bioavailability, and F_{rel} is the relative bioavailability of the complex compared with the pure drug. *Sketch based on Ref. [4].*

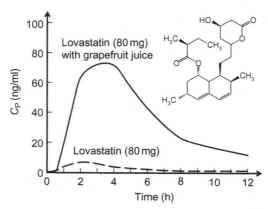

FIGURE 6.4 Plasma concentration time profile of lovastatin after a single oral dose of 80 mg lovastatin taken with and without grapefruit juice. *Sketch based on Ref. [6].*

Lovastatin is an inactive prodrug (see Section 3.4 and Table 3.6), which undergoes enzymatic hydrolysis of a lactone ring to form the active drug lovastatin acid. In a human study, consumption of grapefruit juice resulted in a 15-fold increase in the lovastatin's AUC from 0 to 12 h ($[AUC]_0^{12}$) (Figure 6.4) and a fivefold increase in the $[AUC]_0^{12}$ for lovastatin acid [6]. Thus, consumption of grapefruit and grapefruit juice can result in buildup of lovastatin acid in the body and lead to toxic side effects. Enzyme inhibition can also reduce the oral bioavailability of drugs. St. John's wort is a commonly used herbal medicine. One of its ingredients is the chemical hyperforin, which is an activator of CYP3A4 production. Indinavir, a drug used to treat human immunodeficiency virus (HIV) infection, is relatively well absorbed from the GI tract. It is, however, metabolized by CYP3A4, and drugs, natural products, and excipients that induce CYP3A4 activity can decrease its plasma concentration. Co-administration of St. John's wort reduces the $[AUC]_0^8$ of indinavir by 57% (Figure 6.5). Thus, patients need to be informed about the effects of herbal products such as St. John's wort on the therapeutic efficacy of indinavir.

Some nonionic surfactants used as pharmaceutical excipients, for example, tocopheryl polyethylene glycol succinate (TPGS) and tocopheryl polypropylene glycol succinate (TPPG), are inhibitors of the P-glycoprotein efflux pump and have been tested as enabling pharmaceutical excipients to enhance the oral absorption of drugs such as raloxifene [8]. Raloxifene has very low oral bioavailability (about 2%) because of extensive first-pass effect. Studies in rats have shown that dosing with TPPG increases the bioavailability of raloxifene by about threefold (Figure 6.6). Pharmaceutical formulators can improve the oral bioavailability of certain drugs by employing pharmaceutical excipients that inhibit efflux pumps, for example, P-glycoprotein, which impede drug absorption through the GI mucosa.

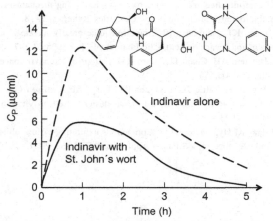

FIGURE 6.5 Plasma concentration time profile of indinavir in healthy volunteers after oral administration of 800 mg of the drug alone and with St. John's wort. *Sketch based on Ref. [7].*

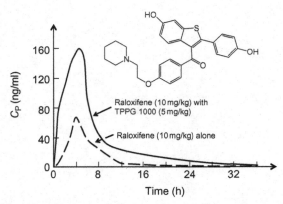

FIGURE 6.6 Plasma concentration time profile of raloxifene in rats after oral administration of the drug given alone and with D-α-tocopheryl polypropylene glycol succinate 1000 (TPPG 1000). *Sketch based on Ref. [9].*

REFERENCES

[1] Axelson JE, Chan GLY, Kirsten EB, Mason WD, Lanman RC, Kerr CR. Food increases the bioavailability of propafenone. Br J Clin Pharmacol 1987;23:735−41.

[2] Neuvonen PJ, Turakka H. Inhibitory effect of various iron salts on absorption of tetracycline in man. Eur J Clin Pharmacol 1974;7:357−60.

[3] Kurkov SV, Loftsson T. Cyclodextrins. Int J Pharmaceut 2013;453:167−80.

[4] Savolainen J, Jarvinen K, Taipale H, Jarho P, Loftsson T, Jarvinen T. Co-administration of a water-soluble polymer increases the usefulness of cyclodextrins in solid oral dosage forms. Pharmaceut Res 1998;15:1696−701.

[5] Bressler R. Grapefruit juice and drug interactions—Exploring mechanisms of this interaction and potential toxicity for certain drugs. Geriatrics 2006;61:12−18.

[6] Kantola T, Kivisto KT, Neuvonen PJ. Grapefruit juice greatly increases serum concentrations of lovastatin and lovastatin acid. Clin Pharmacol Ther 1998;63:397−402.

[7] Piscitelli SC, Burstein AH, Chaitt D, Alfaro RM, Falloon J. Indinavir concentrations and St John's wort. Lancet 2000;355:547−8.

[8] Wempe MF, Wright C, Little JL, Lightner JW, Large SE, Caflisch GB, et al. Inhibiting efflux with novel non-ionic surfactants: rational design based on vitamin E TPGS. Int J Pharmaceut 2009;370:93−102.

[9] Wempe M, Edgar K, Hyatt J, Zima G. Compounds exhibiting efflux inhibitor activity and composition and uses thereof, US Patent Appl. No. 11/730,362, 2007.

Chapter 7

Practice Problems

Chapter Outline

Some of the following problems are based on experimental data extracted from original research publications in international peer-reviewed journals. In all cases, the data have been modified from the original data, and thus do not show the normal experimental variations.

7.1

Scopolamine was administered to 12 healthy men (31.0 ± 4.5 years, 78.2 ± 7.2 kg) as nasal spray (IN), oral tablet (PO), and intravenous (IV) bolus injection [1]. The dose was, in all three cases, 0.40 mg ($D_0 = 0.40$ mg). Blood samples were collected and the plasma scopolamine concentration (C_P) determined at various time points (t).

Time (h)	C_P (pg/ml)[a]		
	IV	IN	PO
0.1	4,500	90	–
0.2	2,650	750	60
0.3	1,900	1,400	80
0.4	1,500	1,240	–
0.5	1,250	1,135	100
0.8	985	1,000	–
1.0	900	900	85
2.0	650	650	60
4.0	360	360	23
5.0	260	260	–
6.0	190	190	–
7.0	138	140	–
8.0	100	100	–

[a]One picogram (pg) is $1.0 \cdot 10^{-9}$ mg or $1.0 \cdot 10^{-12}$ gram (g).

Essential Pharmacokinetics. DOI: http://dx.doi.org/10.1016/B978-0-12-801411-0.00007-X

A. Calculate k, k_{12}, k_{21}, and $t_{1/2}$ after IV bolus administration.
B. Calculate k_a after IN administration.
C. Calculate k and k_a after PO administration.
D. Determine scopolamine bioavailability from the tablets. Determine scopolamine bioavailability from the nasal spray.
E. Determine the total body clearance (Cl_T).
F. On average, 6% of the drug was eliminated unmetabolized in urine after IV administration. Determine the renal clearance (Cl_R).
G. The minimum effective concentration (MEC) is 40 pg/ml. Determine the duration of activity after the IN administration of scopolamine.

7.2

Phenytoin follows nonlinear pharmacokinetics at the therapeutic dosing range. The patient (70 kg) received phenytoin as IV bolus injections at dosing rates (R) of 4.3 and 5.0 mg/kg/day that gave steady-state plasma concentration (C_{SS}) of 8.0 and 20 μg/ml, respectively.

A. Determine V_{max} and K_m in this patient.
B. The therapeutic window of phenytoin is between 10 and 20 μg/ml (see Figure 5.1). Determine the dosing rate that gives a C_{SS} of 15 μg/ml.
C. Determine the Cl_T of phenytoin in this patient when C_{SS} is 15 μg/ml.

7.3

Itraconazole follows the two-compartment open model after administration of oral itraconazole solution [2]. Six healthy male volunteers received itraconazole ($D_0 = 40$ mg) as an oral solution under both fed (○) and fasting (●) conditions. Blood samples were collected and the average itraconazole plasma concentration determined up to 72 h after administration of the drug. The obtained ln C_P versus time profile is shown below.

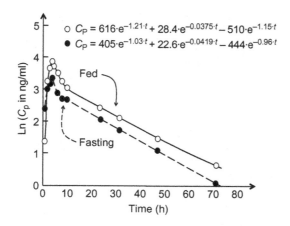

○ $C_P = 616 \cdot e^{-1.21 \cdot t} + 28.4 \cdot e^{-0.0375 \cdot t} - 510 \cdot e^{-1.15 \cdot t}$
● $C_P = 405 \cdot e^{-1.03 \cdot t} + 22.6 \cdot e^{-0.0419 \cdot t} - 444 \cdot e^{-0.96 \cdot t}$

A. Calculate the relative bioavailability (F_{rel}) of the drug administered under the fed condition compared with the drug administered under the fasting condition.

B. How long does it take to reach 90% of C_{av}^{∞} under fed conditions?

C. Common oral dosing schedule for itraconazole is 200 mg every 24 h, and the itraconazole $t_{1/2}$ is most often between 24 and 42 h. This dosing gave average plasma concentration (C_{av}^{∞}) of 1,500 ng/ml. MEC is 500 ng/ml. Determine the onset time when 200 mg itraconazole is administered as an oral solution every 24 h when $t_{1/2}$ is 40 h.

7.4

The figure shows the benoxaprofen plasma concentration in older patients (○) and healthy volunteers (●) after oral administration of 600 mg benoxaprofen [3,4]. Determine the dose regimen for an older patient when a normal patient is administered 600 mg of the drug every 8 h.

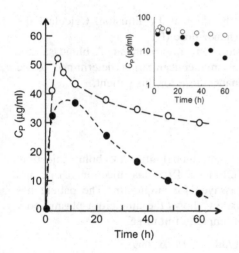

7.5

A birth control vaginal ring contains a combination of etonogestrel and ethinylestradiol [5]. The release rate of etonogestrel from the ring is 120 µg/day, and its bioavailability is 100%. The release rate of ethinylestradiol from the ring is 15 µg/day, and its bioavailability is 55.9%. The sketch below shows the mean plasma concentrations of the two drugs in 16 women after administration of the ring. Estimate the Cl_T for both etonogestrel and ethinylestradiol.

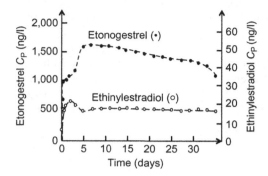

7.6

A drug that follows the one-compartment open model after IV bolus injection has a V_D of 173 ml/kg and a $t_{1/2}$ of 2.0 h. Its therapeutic plasma concentration is 5 µg/ml.

A. A patient (75 kg) is to receive the drug as IV infusion. Calculate the loading dose (D_L) and the maintenance dose (R).

B. After 12 h, the patient did not show any improvement. A blood sample was withdrawn and the drug plasma concentration determined to be 2 µg/ml. Calculate a new maintenance dose for this patient.

7.7

Ampicillin follows the two-compartment model after IV bolus injection. A patient received 570 mg of ampicillin via IV bolus injection. Urine and blood samples were collected and assayed for ampicillin. The patient has normal kidney function. The table below shows the ampicillin plasma concentration and the elimination rate of ampicillin in urine.

Time (h)	C_P (µg/ml)	$\Delta D_U / \Delta t$ (mg)
0.25	30	
1.35	5.5	
2.5	1.7	
4.0	0.671	208
5.0	0.406	123
7.0	0.149	45

A. Calculate A, B, a, b, and $t_{1/2}$.

B. Determine the Cl_T.

C. Calculate the Cl_R. How is ampicillin eliminated after IV bolus injection?

7.8

Sildenafil (M_w 475 daltons [Da]) is used to treat erectile dysfunction. As a free base, sildenafil is a sparingly soluble (0.01 mg/ml water), lipophilic (log $P = 2.5$) drug that permeates the biologic membranes rather easily (H-bond acceptors: 10; H-bond donors: 1). The aqueous solubility of sildenafil citrate is much greater than that of the free base or 4.1 mg/ml, and thus oral dosage forms usually contain sildenafil citrate. The following information was obtained from a pharmacokinetic study of sildenafil citrate, its oral bioavailability, food effects, and dose proportionality in 12−34 healthy male volunteers, and the data shown are the mean values [6].

A. The following profiles were obtained after administration of a single oral dose of sildenafil (25−200 mg) as its citrate salt. Does the drug follow linear pharmacokinetics?

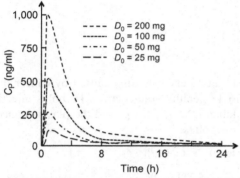

B. The figure below shows the C_P−time profiles of sildenafil after administration of 50 mg of the drug in the form of slow IV infusion and oral tablet. Determine the absolute bioavailability of the tablets. Determine the Cl_T from the IV data. Studies with radiolabeled sildenafil have shown that 92% of the drug is absorbed, although much less intact drug is detected in plasma. Can you explain this difference?

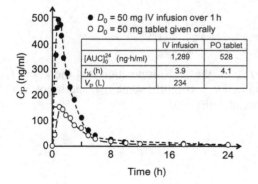

	IV infusion	PO tablet
$[AUC]_0^{24}$ (ng·h/ml)	1,289	528
$t_{1/2}$ (h)	3.9	4.1
V_P (L)	234	

C. The figure below shows the C_P–time profiles of sildenafil after administration of 100 mg of the drug to fasted and fed volunteers. Describe the food effect on the oral bioavailability of sildenafil.

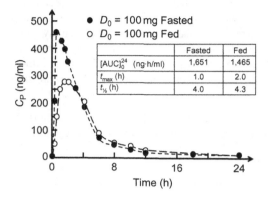

	Fasted	Fed
$[AUC]_0^{24}$ (ng·h/ml)	1,651	1,465
t_{max} (h)	1.0	2.0
$t_{1/2}$ (h)	4.0	4.3

7.9

Ondansetron is used to prevent nausea and vomiting caused by cancer therapy [7]. The drug was given to 18 healthy volunteers as IV bolus injection ($D_{0\ IV} = 8$ mg) and as an oral tablet ($D_{0\ PO} = 8$ mg) and the plasma concentration determined at various time points:

Time (h)	C_p (µg/l) PO	C_p (µg/l) IV
0.6	5.50	
0.8	13.0	
1.0	17.0	38.4
1.5	22.0	
2.0	20.3	29.7
2.5	18.0	
3.0	16.2	23.2
4.0	12.9	18.0
6.0	8.08	11.0
8.0	5.08	6.60
10.0	3.25	4.00
12.0	2.08	2.45

A. Determine the k_a, k, and $t_{1/2}$ for the oral formulation and the k and $t_{1/2}$ for the parenteral formulation. Do you get the same $t_{1/2}$, and if not, why?
B. Calculate the absolute bioavailability (F).
C. Calculate the Cl_T.

7.10

A patient received 1,000 mg of aztreonam via IV bolus injection. Urine was collected and the cumulative amount of aztreonam in urine determined:

Time (h)	D_U (mg)
6	201.6
12	282.6
18	314.4

Determine the first-order elimination rate constant (k) and the fraction of the drug that is excreted unchanged in urine (f_e).

7.11

A newly developed cardiac drug is to be formulated as immediate-release tablets for oral administration. The following pharmacokinetic parameters were obtained during phase I and II studies: the drug follows the one-compartment open model, $t_{1/2} = 30$ h, $V_D = 4.0$ l/kg, $F = 0.80$, the desired therapeutic concentration range is 1.0−2.0 ng/ml, and the minimum toxic concentration (MTC) is 4.0 ng/ml. Determine a dosage regimen for this drug. How much drug should each tablet contain? How frequently should the drug be given? Would you recommend a loading dose?

7.12

Itraconazole is a lipophilic ($\log P = 5.0$) drug that is sparingly soluble in water (about 0.1 µg/ml) and elimination $t_{1/2}$ of 24−42 h. Its plasma protein binding is over 99%. The drug penetrates poorly across the blood−brain barrier, and negligible amounts of the drug dose are excreted unchanged in urine. How does protein binding and lipophilicity affect the terminal $t_{1/2}$ of the drug?

7.13

An antibiotic drug was administered to a patient via IV infusion at 380 mg/h for 6 h. The plasma drug concentration was determined at various time points up to 3 h after the infusion was stopped and a C_P−time profile drawn:

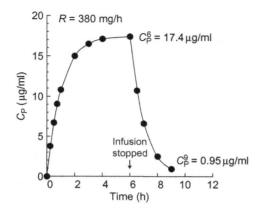

Determine the $t_{1/2}$, V_D, and Cl_T.

7.14

The sketch below shows the plasma concentration versus time profile of a drug ($t_{1/2} = 3.7$ h) given as immediate-release tablets and as sustained-release tablets every 12 h. The dose was adjusted in both cases to give $C_{max}^{\infty} = 15\ \mu g/ml$. What are the advantages of the sustained release tablets?

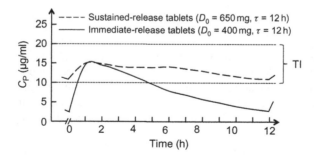

7.15

A patient is on warfarin (an anticoagulant) therapy of one 5-mg tablet a day and is also given cimetidine (a histamine receptor antagonist that inhibits stomach acid production). The warfarin plasma concentration was monitored in the patient (see the sketch below). How would you change the warfarin dosage regimen during co-administration of cimetidine?

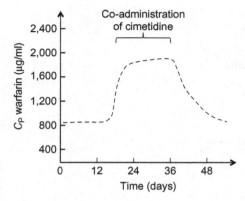

7.16

The effect of kidney function on the pharmacokinetics of acamprosate was investigated after a single drug dose of 666 mg [8]. Blood samples were collected and following semilog plots drawn showing C_P–time plots in three groups: one group with normal kidney function ($Cl_{Cr} > 90$ ml/min), one group with reduced kidney function ($Cl_{Cr} \approx 45$ ml/min), and one group with severely reduced kidney function ($Cl_{Cr} \approx 20$ ml/min). Determine the dosage regimen in a patient with reduced kidney function and in a patient with severely reduced kidney function when a normal adult dose is 666 mg three times a day.

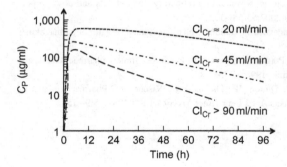

7.17

Clofazimine ($V_D = 7$ l/kg; oral bioavailability 70%) is an antimycobacterial drug that has been used to treat leprosy. The sketch below shows the plasma concentration of the drug in a patient (70 kg) who receives one 50 mg tablet daily [9]. Estimate the biologic $t_{1/2}$ of the drug. Determine the appropriate loading dose (D_L) for this patient.

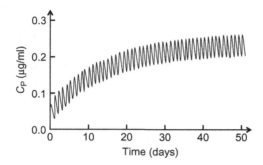

REFERENCES

[1] Putcha L, Tietze KJ, Bourne DWA, Parise CM, Hunter RP, Cintron NM. Bioavailability of intranasal scopolamine in normal subjects. J Pharm Sci US 1996;85:899–902.

[2] Kapsi SG, Ayres JW. Processing factors in development of solid solution formulation of itraconazole for enhancement of drug dissolution and bioavailability. Int J Pharmaceut 2001;229:193–203.

[3] Davies NM, Skjodt NM. Choosing the right nonsteroidal anti-inflammatory drug for the right patient—a pharmacokinetic approach. Clin Pharmacokinet 2000;38:377–92.

[4] Hamdy RC, Murnane B, Perera N, Woodcock K, Koch IM. The pharmacokinetics of benoxaprofen in elderly subjects. Eur J Rheumatol Inflamm 1982;5:69–75.

[5] Timmer CJ, Mulders TMT. Pharmacokinetics of etonogestrel and ethinylestradiol released from a combined contraceptive vaginal ring. Clin Pharmacokinet 2000;39:233–42.

[6] Nichols DJ, Muirhead GJ, Harness JA. Pharmacokinetics of sildenafil citrate after single oral doses in healthy male subjects: absolute bioavailability, food effects and dose proportionality. Br J Clin Pharmacol 2002;53:5S–12S.

[7] Roila F, Delfavero A. Ondansetron clinical pharmacokinetics. Clin Pharmacokinet 1995;29:95–109.

[8] Saivin S, Hulot T, Chabac S, Potgieter A, Durbin P, Houin G. Clinical pharmacokinetics of acamprosate. Clin Pharmacokinet 1998;35:331–45.

[9] Schaad-Lanyi Z, Dieterle W, Dubois JP, Theobald W, Vischer W. Pharmacokinetics of clofazimine in healthy volunteers. Int J Lepr Other Mycobact Dis 1987;55:9–15.

Appendix I

Answers to Problems in Chapter 7

7.1

You should plot the data yourself.

A

The C_P versus time plotted indicates that scopolamine follows the two-compartment open model after IV bolus injection (see Example 2.4). The plot follows Eq. (2.35):

$$C_P = Ae^{-a \cdot t} + Be^{-b \cdot t}$$

t (h)	C_P (pg/ml)	ln C_P	C'_P (pg/ml)	ln($C_P - C'_P$)	
0.1	4,500	8.412	1,195	8.103	ln($C_P - C'_P$) = ln$A$ − $a \cdot t$
0.2	2,650	7.882	1,158	7.308	Slope = − 6.918 h^{-1} = − a
0.3	1,900	7.550	1,122	6.657	a = 6.92 h^{-1}
0.4	1,500	7.313	1,088	6.021	Intercept = 8.750 = ln$A$
0.5	1,250	7.131	1,054	5.278	A = 6308 pg/ml
0.8	985	6.893	960	3.219	Correlation = 0.9997
1.0	900	6.802			
2.0	650	6.477			lnC'_P = ln$B$ − $b \cdot t$
4.0	360	5.886			Slope = − 0.3125 h^{-1} = − b
5.0	260	5.561			b = 0.313 h^{-1}
6.0	190	5.247			Intercept = 7.1168 = ln$B$
7.0	138	4.927			B = 1233 pg/ml
8.0	100	4.605			Correlation = 1.000

$A = 6{,}308$ pg/ml; $B = 1{,}233$ pg/ml; $a = 6.92\ \text{h}^{-1}$; $b = 0.313\ \text{h}^{-1}$

$C_P = 6308 \cdot e^{-6.92 \cdot t} + 1233 \cdot e^{-0.313 \cdot t}$, where C_P is in pg/ml and t in hours.
Then, k, k_{12}, k_{21}, and $t_{1/2}$ can be calculated:

$$k = \frac{a \cdot b \cdot (A + B)}{A \cdot b + B \cdot a} = \frac{6.92 \cdot 0.313 \cdot (6308 + 1233)}{6308 \cdot 0.313 + 1233 \cdot 6.92} = 1.55\ \text{h}^{-1}$$

$$k_{12} = \frac{A \cdot B \cdot (b-a)^2}{(A + B) \cdot (A \cdot b + B \cdot a)} = \frac{6308 \cdot 1233 \cdot (0.313 - 6.92)^2}{(6308 + 1233) \cdot (6308 \cdot 0.313 + 1233 \cdot 6.92)}$$

$$= 4.28\ \text{h}^{-1}$$

$$k_{21} = \frac{A \cdot b + B \cdot a}{A + B} = \frac{6308 \cdot 0.313 + 1233 \cdot 6.92}{6308 + 1233} = 1.39\ \text{h}^{-1}$$

$$t_{1/2} = \frac{\ln 2}{b} = \frac{0.693}{0.313} = 2.2\ \text{h}$$

We can use the following two equations (Eqs. (2.35) and (2.36)) to check the results:

$$a + b = k_{12} + k_{21} + k \Rightarrow 6.92 + 0.313 = 4.28 + 1.39 + 1.55 \Rightarrow 7.23 \approx 7.22$$

$$a \cdot b = k_{21} \cdot k \Rightarrow 6.92 \cdot 0.313 = 1.39 \cdot 1.55 \Rightarrow 2.17 \approx 2.16$$

B

The C_P versus time plotted indicates that scopolamine follows the two-compartment open model with first-order absorption after IN administration (see Example 2.8). The plot follows Eq. (2.79):

$$C_P = Ae^{-a \cdot t} + Be^{-b \cdot t} - Ce^{-k_a \cdot t}$$

t (h)	C_P (pg/ml)	ln C_P	C_p' (pg/ml)	$(C_P - C_p')$	$\ln(C_P - C_p')$	C_p'' $(C_P - C_p')$	$(C_p'' - (C_P - C_p'))$	$\ln(C_p'' - (C_P - C_p'))$
0.1	90		1,212	−1122		1,048	2,170	7.682
0.2	750		1,175	−425		572	952	6.859
0.3	1,400		1,139	261	5.565			
0.4	1,240		1,103	137	4.920			
0.5	1,135		1,069	66	4.190			
0.8	1,000	6.908						
1.0	900	6.802						
2.0	650	6.477						
4.0	360	5.886						
5.0	260	5.561						
6.0	190	5.247						
7.0	140	4.942						
8.0	100	4.605						

$C_p'' - (C_P - C_p') = C \cdot e^{-k_a \cdot t}$ or
$\ln(C_p'' - (C_P - C_p')) = \ln C - k_a \cdot t$
Slope $= -k_a = -8.23\ \text{h}^{-1}$
$k_a = -8.23\ \text{h}^{-1}$
Intercept $= 8.505 = \ln C$
$C = 4939$ pg/ml

$C_p' = B \cdot e^{-b \cdot t}$ or
$\ln C_p' = \ln B - b \cdot t$
Slope $= -b = -0.314\ \text{h}^{-1}$
$b = 0.314\ \text{h}^{-1}$
Intercept $= \ln B = 7.1318$
$B = 1251$ pg/ml
Correlation $= 1.000$

$C_p' = (C_P - C_p') = A \cdot e^{-a \cdot t}$ or
$\ln C_p' - \ln(C_P - C_p') = \ln A - a \cdot t$
Slope $= -a = -6.875\ \text{h}^{-1}$
$\ln A = 7.642$
$A = 2083$ pg/ml
Correlation $= 0.999$

$k_a = 8.23\ \text{h}^{-1}$ and the half-life of the absorption is $t_{1/2} = \ln 2/k_a = 0.693/8.23 = 0.084\ \text{h} = 5.1\ \text{min}$.

C

The C_P versus time plotted indicates that scopolamine follows the one-compartment open model with first-order absorption after PO administration (see Example 2.6). The plot follows Eq. (2.70):

$$C_P = Be^{-k \cdot t} - Ae^{-k_a \cdot t}$$

t (h)	C_P (pg/ml)	ln C_P	C_P'(pg/ml)	$(C_P - C_P')$	$ln(C_P - C_P')$
0.2	60		119	59	4.078
0.3	80		114	34	3.526
0.5	100	4.605			
1.0	85	4.443			
2.0	60	4.094			
4.0	23	3.135			

For the first two rows:
$$\begin{cases} \ln(C_P - C_P') = \ln B - k \cdot t \\ \text{Slope} = -k_a = -5.52 \text{ h}^{-1} \\ k = 5.52 \text{ h}^{-1} \\ \text{Intercept} = \ln B = 5.182 \\ B = 178 \text{ pg/ml} \end{cases}$$

For the remaining rows:
$$\begin{cases} \ln C_P' = \ln B - k \cdot t \\ \text{Slope} = -k = -0.424 \text{ h}^{-1} \\ k = 0.424 \text{ h}^{-1} \\ \text{Intercept} = \ln B = 4.864 \\ B = 130 \text{ pg/ml} \\ \text{Correlation} = 0.996 \end{cases}$$

$k = 0.42 \text{ h}^{-1}$ and $k_a = 5.52 \text{ h}^{-1}$ $t_{1/2} = \ln 2/k_a = 0.693/5.52 = 0.13$ h $= 7.5$ min

The drug is absorbed about 50% faster from the nasal cavity than from the GI tract.

D

Equations. (2.51), (2.84), and (2.85) are applied (see Example 2.9):

$$IV{:}[AUC]_0^\infty = \frac{A}{a} + \frac{B}{b} = \frac{6,308 \text{ pg/ml}}{6.92 \text{ h}^{-1}} + \frac{1,233 \text{ pg/ml}}{0.313 \text{ h}^{-1}} = 4,851 \text{ pg} \cdot \text{h/ml}$$

$$PO{:} [AUC]_0^\infty = \frac{A}{k} - \frac{B}{k_a} = \frac{130 \text{ pg/ml}}{0.424 \text{ h}^{-1}} - \frac{178 \text{ pg/ml}}{5.52 \text{ h}^{-1}} = 274 \text{ pg} \cdot \text{h/ml}$$

$$IN{:} [AUC]_0^\infty = \frac{A}{a} + \frac{B}{b} - \frac{C}{k_a} = \frac{2,083 \text{ pg/ml}}{6.875 \text{ h}^{-1}} + \frac{1,251 \text{ pg/ml}}{0.314 \text{ h}^{-1}} - \frac{4,939 \text{ pg/ml}}{8.23 \text{ h}^{-1}}$$

$$= 3,687 \text{ pg} \cdot \text{h/ml}$$

Then you apply Eq. (2.80) to determine the bioavailability ($D_{IV} = D_{PO} = D_{IN} = 0.4$ mg):

$$F_{PO} = \frac{[AUC]_{PO}/Dose_{PO}}{[AUC]_{IV}/Dose_{IV}} = \frac{[AUC]_{PO}}{[AUC]_{IV}} = \frac{274}{4851} = 0.056 \text{ or } 5.6\%$$

$$F_{IN} = \frac{[AUC]_{IN}}{[AUC]_{IV}} = \frac{3687}{4851} = 0.76 \text{ or } 76\%$$

E

You should use the IV values to calculate the Cl_T (Eqs. (2.45) and (2.47)):

$$Cl_T = k \cdot V_P = b \cdot (V_D)_{area} = \frac{D_0}{[AUC]_0^\infty} = \frac{4 \cdot 10^8 \text{ pg}}{4,851(\text{pg} \cdot \text{h/ml})} = 82,457 \text{ ml/h}$$

$$= 1,374 \text{ ml/min}$$

F

Fraction excreted unchanged in urine: $f_e = k_e/k = 0.06$ or 6%. From Eq. (2.97):

$$Cl_R = Cl_T \cdot \frac{k_e}{k} = 1,374 \text{ ml/min} \cdot 0.06 = 82 \text{ ml/min}$$

G

C_P reaches 40 pg/ml within 6 min after IN administration. Then you calculate at what time C_P goes below 40 pg/ml:

$$C'_P = B \cdot e^{-b \cdot t} \text{ or } \ln C'_P = \ln B - b \cdot t \Rightarrow t = \frac{\ln B/C'_P}{b} = \frac{\ln 1,251/40}{0.314 \text{ h}^{-1}} = 11 \text{ h}$$

The duration is approximately 11 h.

7.2

A

At steady-state, the dosing rate (R) is to drug elimination from the body $(- dC_p/dt)$, or at steady-state $R = - dC_{SS}/dt$, and Eq. (2.151) can be written as:

$$R = - \frac{dC_{SS}}{dt} = \frac{V_{max} C_{SS}}{K_m + C_{SS}}$$

This equation can be rearranged to give:

$$R = V_{max} - K_m \cdot \frac{R}{C_{SS}}$$

Inserting the values gives (i) $4,300 = V_{max} - K_m \cdot 537.5$ and (ii) $5,000 = V_{max} - K_m \cdot 250$. Solving these two equations together gives $V_{max} = 5.6$ mg/kg/day and $K_m = 2.4 \text{ μg/ml} = 2.4$ mg/l.

B

For this 70 kg patient, the V_{max} is 382 mg/day:

$$R = \frac{V_{max} C_{SS}}{K_m + C_{SS}} = \frac{382 \text{ mg/day} \cdot 15 \text{ mg/l}}{2.4 \text{ mg/l} + 15 \text{ mg/l}} = 329 \text{ mg/day}$$

C

According to Eq. (2.95), Cl_T is defined as rate of drug elimination divided by the plasma drug concentration or at steady-state:

$$Cl_T = \frac{\text{rate of elimination}}{\text{plasma concentration}} = \frac{R}{C_{SS}} = \frac{329 \text{ mg/day}}{15 \text{ mg/l}} = 21.9 \text{ l/day} = 15.2 \text{ ml/min}$$

7.3

A

The C_P versus time profiles are fitted to Eq. (2.79), the equation for the two-compartment model with first-order absorption:

$$C_P = Ae^{-a \cdot t} + Be^{-b \cdot t} - Ce^{-k_a \cdot t}$$

The AUC is calculated from Eq. (2.85):

Fed: $[AUC]_0^\infty = \dfrac{A}{a} + \dfrac{B}{b} - \dfrac{C}{k_a} = \dfrac{616}{1.21} + \dfrac{28.4}{0.0375} - \dfrac{510}{1.15} = 822.9 \text{ ng} \cdot \text{h/ml}$

Fasting: $[AUC]_0^\infty = \dfrac{A}{a} + \dfrac{B}{b} - \dfrac{C}{k_a} = \dfrac{405}{1.03} + \dfrac{22.6}{0.0419} - \dfrac{444}{0.96} = 470.1 \text{ ng} \cdot \text{h/ml}$

And then the relative bioavailability is calculated according to Eq. (2.86), where $\text{Dose}_A = \text{Dose}_B$:

$$F_{rel} = \frac{[AUC]_A/\text{Dose}_A}{[AUC]_B/\text{Dose}_B} = \frac{822.9}{470.1} = 1.75 \quad \text{(the bioavailability is increased}$$

by 75%)

B

Equation (2.128) is applied assuming that $k_a \gg b$ (i.e., the IV equation can be applied):

$$n \cdot \tau = \frac{\ln(1 - f_{ss})}{-k} \approx \frac{\ln(1 - f_{ss})}{-b} = \frac{\ln(1 - 0.90)}{-0.0375 \text{ h}^{-1}} = 61.4 \text{ h} \approx 3 \text{ days}$$

C

500 ng/ml is 33.3% of C_{av}^{∞}:

$$n \cdot \tau = \frac{\ln(1 - f_{ss})}{-k} = \frac{\ln(1 - f_{ss})}{-0.693} \cdot t_{\frac{1}{2}} = \frac{\ln(1 - 0.333)}{-0.693} \cdot 40\,h \approx 24\,h$$

The onset time is the time right after administration of the second dose.

7.4

First-order elimination is observed from 12 h. Estimation of the elimination rate constant from the figure:

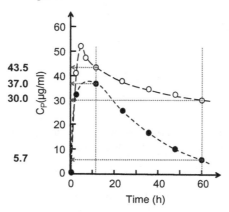

Then, the first-order rate equation (Eq. (2.6)) is used to calculate the rate constants for older patients (k') and healthy volunteers (k):

$$\ln C_P = \ln C_P^0 - k \cdot t \Rightarrow k = \frac{\ln\left(C_P^0 / C_P\right)}{t}$$

Heathy volunteers: $k = \dfrac{\ln(37/5.7)}{48} = 3.90 \cdot 10^{-2}\,h^{-1}$

Older patients: $k' = \dfrac{\ln(43.5/30)}{48} = 7.74 \cdot 10^{-3}\,h^{-1}$

Then, we can use Eq. (5.4) to calculate the new dose:

$$D_0' = D_0 \cdot \frac{k'}{k} = 600\,mg \cdot \frac{7.74 \cdot 10^{-3}\,h^{-1}}{3.90 \cdot 10^{-2}\,h^{-1}} \approx 120\,mg \text{ given every 8 h.}$$

We can also keep the dose the same but change τ (Eq. (5.5)):

$$\tau' = \tau \cdot \frac{k}{k'} = 8 \cdot \frac{3.90 \cdot 10^{-2}\,h^{-1}}{7.74 \cdot 10^{-3}\,h^{-1}} = 40\,h \text{ , which is not realistic (τ has to be}$$
≤ 24 h, e.g., 6, 8, 12, or 24 h).

Or we can change both τ and D_0 to maintain C_{av}^{∞} constant (Eq. (5.6)):

$$\frac{D_0'}{\tau'} = \frac{k'}{k} \cdot \frac{D_0}{\tau} \Rightarrow \frac{D_0'}{\tau'} = \frac{7.74 \cdot 10^{-3} \text{ h}^{-1}}{3.90 \cdot 10^{-2} \text{ h}^{-1}} \cdot \frac{600 \text{ mg}}{8 \text{ h}} \Rightarrow \frac{D_0'}{\tau'}$$

$$= \frac{7.74 \cdot 10^{-3} \text{ h}^{-1}}{3.90 \cdot 10^{-2} \text{ h}^{-1}} \cdot \frac{600 \text{ mg}}{8 \text{ h}} = 14.9$$

If $\tau = 24$, then $D_0' = 24 \cdot 14.9 \approx 360$ mg
If $\tau = 12$, then $D_0' = 12 \cdot 14.9 \approx 180$ mg

7.5

Equations (2.23) and (2.95) are used to calculate Cl_T. At steady-state, the rate of drug delivery from the vagina is equal to the rate of drug elimination $(-dD_{Vag}/dt = dD_E/dt)$. The delivery rate is equal to the drug release rate from the vaginal ring times the bioavailability:

$$Cl_T = \frac{F \cdot R}{C_{SS}}$$

From the figure, the C_{SS} for etonogestrel is estimated to be 1,500 ng/l and that for ethinylestradiol to be 18 ng/l.

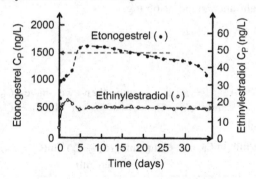

Etonogestrel: $Cl_T = \dfrac{F \cdot R}{C_{SS}} \approx \dfrac{1.00 \cdot 120 \text{ μg/day}}{1.50 \text{ μg/l}} = 80 \text{ l/day}$

$$= 3.3 \text{ l/h} = 56 \text{ ml/min}$$

Ethinylestradiol: $Cl_T = \dfrac{F \cdot R}{C_{SS}} \approx \dfrac{0.559 \cdot 15 \text{ μg/day}}{0.018 \text{ μg/l}} = 466 \text{ l/day}$

$$= 19.4 \text{ l/h} = 323 \text{ ml/min}$$

7.6

A

Equation (2.23) is applied to calculate the maintenance dose (R):

$$C_{SS} = \frac{R}{V_D \cdot k} \Rightarrow R = C_{SS} \cdot V_D \cdot k = C_{SS} \cdot V_D \cdot \frac{\ln 2}{t_{1/2}}$$

$$= 5 \text{ ml}/1 \cdot 0.173 \text{ l/kg} \cdot 75 \text{ kg} \cdot \frac{\ln 2}{2 \text{ h}} = 22.5 \text{ mg/h}$$

Equation (2.24) is applied to determine the loading dose:

$$D_L = V_D \cdot C_{SS} = 0.173 \text{ l/kg} \cdot 75 \text{ kg} \cdot 5 \text{ mg/l} = 65 \text{ mg}$$

B

We assume that C_{SS} is lower than anticipated due to faster excretion.

$$C_{SS} = \frac{R}{V_D \cdot k} \Rightarrow 2.0 \text{ mg/l} = \frac{22.5 \text{ mg/h}}{0.173 \text{ l/kg} \cdot 75 \text{ kg} \cdot k} \Rightarrow k = 0.867 \text{ h}^{-1} \Rightarrow t_{1/2} = 0.8 \text{ h}$$

C_{SS} has been reached after 12 h ($= 15$ half-lives).

$$R = C_{SS} \cdot V_D \cdot k = C_{SS} \cdot V_D \cdot k = 5 \text{ ml}/1 \cdot 0.173 \text{ l/kg} \cdot 75 \text{ kg} \cdot 0.867 \text{ h}^{-1} = 56.2 \text{ mg/h}$$

D_L will remain unchanged or 65 mg.

7.7

A

Eq. (2.34): $C_P = A e^{-a \cdot t} + B e^{-b \cdot t}$, and then we have $C_P' = B \cdot e^{-b \cdot t}$ or $\ln C_P' = \ln B - b \cdot t$ and $C_P - C_P' = A \cdot e^{-a \cdot t}$ or $\ln(C_P - C_P') = \ln A - a \cdot t$ (see Example 2.4).

Time (h)	C_P (μg/ml)	$\ln C_P$	C_P'(μg/ml)	$(C_P - C_P')$ (μg/ml)	$\ln(C_P - C_P')$
0.25	30	3.4011	4.40	25.6	3.2426
1.35	5.5	1.7047	2.53	2.97	1.0886
2.5	1.7	0.5306	1.42	0.28	-1.2730
4.0	0.671	-0.3990			
5.0	0.406	-0.9014			
7.0	0.149	-1.9038			

Slope $= -b = -0,5015 \text{ h}^{-1} \Rightarrow b = 0,502 \text{ h}^{-1}$
Intercept $= \ln B = 1,6068 \Rightarrow B = 5,0 \text{ }\mu\text{g/ml}$

Slope $= -a = -2,0073 \text{ h}^{-1} \Rightarrow a = 2,01 \text{ h}^{-1}$
Intercept $= \ln A = 3,763 \Rightarrow A = 43,1 \text{ }\mu\text{g/ml}$

$A = 43.1 \text{ }\mu\text{g/ml}; \; a = 2.01 \text{ h}^{-1}$
$B = 5.0 \text{ }\mu\text{g/ml}; \; b = 0.502 \text{ h}^{-1} \quad t_{1/2} = \frac{\ln 2}{b} = \frac{0.693}{0.502 \text{ h}^{-1}} = 1.4 \text{ h}$

B

From Eq. (2.38): $k = \dfrac{a \cdot b \cdot (A + B)}{A \cdot b + B \cdot a} = \dfrac{2.01\ \text{h}^{-1} \cdot 0.502\ \text{h}^{-1} \cdot (43.1 + 5.0)\mu\text{g/ml}}{43.1\ \mu\text{g/ml} \cdot 0.502\ \text{h}^{-1} + 5.0\ \mu\text{g/ml} \cdot 2.01\ \text{h}^{-1}} = 1.53\ \text{h}^{-1}$

From Eq. (2.43): $V_P = \dfrac{D_0}{A + B} = \dfrac{570\ \text{mg}}{(43.1 + 5.0)\text{mg/l}} = 11.9\ \text{l}$

From Eq. (2.45): $\text{Cl}_T = k \cdot V_P = 1.53\ \text{h}^{-1} \cdot 11.9\ \text{l} = 18.2\ \text{l/h} = 303\ \text{ml/min}$

C

Eq. (2.99):

$$\text{Cl}_R = \frac{\text{rate of excretion}}{\text{plasma concentration}} = \frac{\text{filtration rate} + \text{secretion rate} - \text{reabsorption rate}}{C_P}$$

$$= \frac{dD_U/dt}{C_P}$$

$$\text{Cl}_R = \frac{dD_U/dt}{C_P} = \frac{203\ \mu\text{g/min}}{0.671\ \mu\text{g/ml}} = \frac{123\ \mu\text{g/min}}{0.406\ \mu\text{g/ml}} = \frac{45\ \mu\text{g/min}}{0.149\ \mu\text{g/ml}} = 303\ \text{ml/min}$$

$\text{Cl}_T = \text{Cl}_R = 303$ ml/min. According to this, ampicillin is only excreted unchanged in urine. However, clinical handbooks tell us that about 90% (not 100%) of parenterally administered ampicillin is excreted unchanged in urine.

$\text{Cl}_R/\text{Cl}_{Cr} \approx 2.5$ or much greater than unity, and thus the drug is excreted by glomerular filtration as well as by tubular excretion (see Section 2.6.2).

7.8

A

Equation (2.83) states that for linear pharmacokinetics $[\text{AUC}]_0^\infty \propto D_0$:

$$[\text{AUC}]_0^\infty = \frac{F \cdot D_0}{V_D \cdot k} = \left(\frac{F}{V_D \cdot k}\right) \cdot D_0 \quad \text{or} \quad C_{\max} \approx \text{constant} \cdot D_0$$

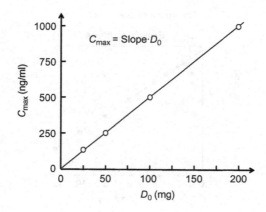

Linear relationship indicates that the pharmacokinetics is linear up to at least $D_0 = 200$ mg.

B

The absolute bioavailability (F) is defined by Eq. (2.80). Since the oral and IV doses are equal, we can calculate F as follows:

$$F = \frac{[AUC]_0^{24}{}_{PO}}{[AUC]_0^{24}{}_{IV}} = \frac{528 \text{ ng} \cdot \text{h/ml}}{1,289 \text{ ng} \cdot \text{h/ml}} = 0.41 \text{ or } 41\%$$

The absolute bioavailability is 41%, but studies with radiolabeled sildenafil show 92% oral availability. This indicates extensive first-pass metabolism. The drug displays high pharmaceutical availability (F_{pharm}) or 92%, but low biologic availability (F_{bio}) (see Section 1.1 and Eqs. (1.1) and (1.2)).

$$F = F_{pharm} \times F_{bio} \Rightarrow 0.41 = 0.92 \times F_{bio} \Rightarrow F_{bio} = \frac{0.41}{0.92} = 0.45 \text{ or } 45\%$$

C

Food slows sildenafil absorption from the GI tract increasing t_{max} from 1 to 2 h and reducing C_{max} from about 460 ng/ml to about 280 ng/ml. The bioavailability of sildenafil is reduced a little, or by about 12%. The main difference is doubling of t_{max}. Thus, if the patient has eaten a large meal, it will take the drug longer to display its therapeutic effect.

7.9

A

Equation (2.66) or (2.70) is applied for the PO pharmacokinetics. The semilog plot shows that the absorption phase is from 0 to 1.5 h and the elimination phase from 2.0 h:

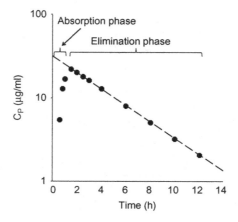

PO:

Time (h)	C_P (µg/l)	ln C_P	C_P'(µg/l)	$(C_P' - C_P)$ (µg/l)	ln($C_P' - C_P$)	
0.6	5.50	1.705	27.63	22.13	3.097	Slope $= -k_a = -2.473$ h^{-1}
0.8	13.0	2.565	26.43	13.42	2.597	$k_a = 2.47$ h^{-1}
1.0	17.0	2.833	25.23	13.42	2.108	ln $A = 4.579$
						$A = 97.42$ µg/l
1.5	22.0	3.091				
2.0	20.3	3.011				
2.5	18.0	2.890				Slope $= -k = -0.227$ h^{-1}
3.0	16.2	2.785				$k = 0.227$ h^{-1}
4.0	12.9	2.557				$t_{1/2} = \ln2/k = 3.01$ h
6.0	8.08	2.086				ln $B = 3.456$
8.0	5.08	1.625				$B = 31.69$ µg/l
10.0	3.25	1.179				
12.0	2.08	0.732				

$$C_P = Be^{-k \cdot t} - Ae^{-k_a \cdot t} = 31.7\ \mu g/l \cdot e^{-0.227\ h^{-1} \cdot t} - 97.4\ \mu g/l \cdot e^{-2.47\ h^{-1} \cdot t}$$

IV:

Time (h)	C_P (µg/l)	ln C_P	
1.0	38.4	3.648	
2.0	29.7	3.391	
3.0	23.2	3.144	Slope $= -k = -0.250$ h^{-1}
4.0	18.0	2.890	$k = 0.250$ h^{-1}
6.0	11.0	2.398	$t_{1/2} = \ln2/k = 2.77$ h
8.0	6.60	1.887	ln $C_P^0 = 3.894$
10.0	4.00	1.386	$C_P^0 = 49.1$ µg/L
12.0	2.45	0.896	

$$C_P = \frac{D_0}{V_D} \cdot e^{-k \cdot t} = C_P^0 \cdot e^{-k \cdot t} \Rightarrow C_P = 49.1\ \mu g/l \cdot e^{-0.250\ h^{-1} \cdot t}$$

Figure 2.14 shows that drug is still being absorbed in the elimination phase and especially in the beginning of the phase. Thus, the slope of the elimination phase after oral absorption is less than that observed after IV bolus injection. Consequently, the observed $t_{1/2}$ after oral administration becomes smaller than the $t_{1/2}$ observed after IV bolus injection. The $t_{1/2}$ value determined from the IV data is more accurate than that determined from the oral data.

B

IV (Eq. (2.82)): $[AUC]_0^\infty = \dfrac{D_0}{V_D \cdot k} = \dfrac{C_P^0}{k} = \dfrac{49.1\ \mu g/l}{0.250\ h^{-1}} = 196.4\ \mu g \cdot h/l$

PO (Eq. (2.84)): $[AUC]_0^\infty = \dfrac{B}{k} - \dfrac{A}{k_a} = \dfrac{31.7\ \mu g/l}{0.227\ h^{-1}} - \dfrac{97.4\ \mu g/l}{2.47\ h^{-1}} = 98.34\ \mu g \cdot h/l$

$F = \dfrac{[AUC]_{0\ PO}^{24}}{[AUC]_{0\ IV}^{24}} = \dfrac{98.34\ \mu g \cdot h/l}{196.4\ \mu g \cdot h/l} = 0.50\ \text{or}\ 50\%$

C

Equation (2.4): $V_D = \dfrac{D_0}{C_P^0} = \dfrac{8{,}000\ \mu g}{49.1\ \mu g/l} = 163\ l$

Equation (2.8): $Cl_T = V_D \cdot k = 163\ l \cdot 0.250\ h^{-1} = 40.7\ l/h = 679\ ml/min$

7.10

Equation (2.19): $\ln\left(\dfrac{dD_U}{dt}\right) = \ln(k_e \cdot D_0) - k \cdot t$ or $\ln\left(\dfrac{\Delta D_U}{\Delta t}\right) = \ln(k_e \cdot D_0) - k \cdot t$

Prepare the data to be plotted according to Eq. (2.19).

Period (h)	ΔD_u (mg)	$\Delta D_u/\Delta t$ (mg/h)	t_m (h)	$\ln(\Delta D_u/\Delta t)$
0–6	201.6	33.2	3	3.503
6–12	81.0	13.5	9	2.603
12–18	31.8	5.3	15	1.668

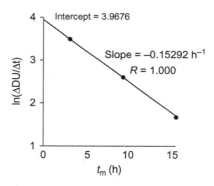

$\text{Intercept} = \ln(k_e \cdot D_0) = 3.9676 \Rightarrow (k_e \cdot D_0) = 52.86\ mg/h \Rightarrow k_e = 5.29 \cdot 10^{-2}\ h^{-1}$

$\text{Slope} = -k = -0.15292\ h^{-1} \Rightarrow k = 0.153\ h^{-1}$

$f_e = \dfrac{k_e}{k} = \dfrac{5.29 \cdot 10^{-2}\ h^{-1}}{0.153\ h^{-1}} = 0.346$ or 34.6% $\left(f_e = \dfrac{D_U^\infty}{D_0} > \dfrac{D_U^{18}}{D_0} = 0.314\right)$

7.11

The drug has long $t_{1/2}$, and we do not have the information about the absorption rate constants. Thus, we use the IV equations, assuming that $k_a \gg k$.

It takes one $t_{1/2}$ for C_P to decrease from 2 to 1 ng/or 30 h. If the drug is given once a day (q.d.), and if we set $C_{av}^{\infty} = 1.5$ ng/ml, then (Eq. (2.135)):

$$C_{av}^{\infty} = \frac{F \cdot D_0}{V_D \cdot k \cdot \tau} \quad \text{or} \quad 1.5\,\mu g/l = \frac{0.80 \cdot D_0}{4\,l/kg \cdot (\ln 2/30\,h) \cdot 24\,h} \Rightarrow D_0 = 4.16\,\mu g/kg$$

Then, C_{max}^{∞} and C_{min}^{∞} need to be determined (modified Eqs. (2.120) and (2.121)):

$$C_{max}^{\infty} = \frac{F \cdot D_0}{V_D} \cdot \left(\frac{1}{1 - e^{-k \cdot \tau}}\right) = \frac{0.80 \cdot 4.16\,\mu g/kg}{4.0\,l/kg} \cdot \left(\frac{1}{1 - e^{-(\ln 2/30\,h) \cdot 24\,h}}\right)$$

$$= 1.95\,\mu g/l = 1.95\,ng/ml$$

$$C_{min}^{\infty} = \frac{F \cdot D_0}{V_D} \cdot \left(\frac{1}{1 - e^{-k \cdot \tau}}\right) \cdot e^{-k \cdot \tau} = C_{max}^{\infty} \cdot e^{-k \cdot \tau} = 1.95\,ng/ml \cdot e^{-(\ln 2/30\,h) \cdot 24\,h}$$

$$= 1.12\,ng/ml$$

D_0 should be 0.20, 0.30 and 0.40 mg, for 50-, 70-, and 100-kg patients, respectively. If a 50-kg patient receives a 0.30-mg tablet once a day, then C_{max}^{∞} will be 2.9 µg/ml, which is below the MTC, but a 100-kg patient receiving a 0.30-mg tablet once a day will have C_{min}^{∞} of 0.8 ng/ml. Thus, it might be better to give 2 mg/kg twice a day (b.i.d.):

$$C_{max}^{\infty} = \frac{F \cdot D_0}{V_D} \cdot \left(\frac{1}{1 - e^{-k \cdot \tau}}\right) = \frac{0.80 \cdot 2.0\,\mu g/kg}{4.0\,l/kg} \cdot \left(\frac{1}{1 - e^{-(\ln 2/30\,h) \cdot 12\,h}}\right)$$

$$= 1.65\,\mu g/l = 1.65\,ng/ml$$

$$C_{min}^{\infty} = \frac{F \cdot D_0}{V_D} \cdot \left(\frac{1}{1 - e^{-k \cdot \tau}}\right) \cdot e^{-k \cdot \tau} = C_{max}^{\infty} \cdot e^{-k \cdot \tau} = 1.65\,ng/ml \cdot e^{-(\ln 2/30\,h) \cdot 12\,h}$$

$$= 1.25\,ng/ml$$

In that case, D_0 should be 0.10, 0.14, and 0.20 mg, for 50-, 70-, and 100-kg patients, respectively. If each tablet contains 0.15 mg of the drug twice a day, then C_{max}^{∞} will be about 2.5 µg/ml, which is below the MTC, but a 100-kg patient receiving a 0.15-mg tablet twice a day will have C_{min}^{∞} of about 0.9 ng/ml. Alternatively, the 100-kg patient could be given 1½ tablets twice a day and the 50-kg patient one tablet in the morning but ½ tablet in the evening. For a "normal" 70-kg patient: $D_0 = 0.15$ mg and $\tau = 12$ h.

The therapeutic concentration is rather narrow, and the half-life of the drug is long. Thus, it takes a long time for the drug to reach the MEC.

If $t_{1/2}$ is 30 h it takes over 4 days for the drug plasma concentration to reach 90% of its steady-state value (Eq. (2.127)):

$$n \cdot t = \frac{\ln(1 - f_{ss})}{-k} = \frac{\ln(1 - f_{ss})}{-0.693} \cdot t_{1/2} = \frac{\ln 0.10}{-0.693} \cdot 30\,h \approx 100\,h \text{ or more than 4 days}$$

A loading dose should be given. Equation (2.130) can be applied to calculate the loading dose:

$$D_L = D_0 \cdot \frac{1}{1 - e^{-k \cdot \tau}} = 0.15 \cdot \frac{1}{1 - e^{-(\ln 2/30\,h) \cdot 12\,h}} = 0.47\,mg$$

Thus, D_L is three 0.15-mg tablets.

7.12

Drug molecules bound to plasma proteins are not excreted in urine via glomerular filtration (i.e., permeation through semipermeable membrane that is impermeable to the large protein molecules), only the unbound drug molecules are excreted. Protein binding reduces the ability of drug molecules to permeate biologic membranes such as the blood−brain barrier. Furthermore, drug molecules bound to plasma proteins are generally protected against enzymatic degradation. Due to its lipophilicity, itraconazole partitions from aqueous plasma into fat tissue, where it is also protected against enzymatic degradation. In general, lipophilic and highly ($>99\%$) protein-bound drugs have longer terminal half-life compared with the more hydrophilic drugs that display somewhat lower protein binding.

7.13

Equation (2.6): $\ln C_P = \ln C_P^0 - k \cdot t \Rightarrow \ln 0.95 = \ln 17.4 - k \cdot 3\,h \Rightarrow k = 0.97\,h^{-1}$

$$t_{1/2} = \frac{\ln 2}{k} = \frac{0.693}{0.97\,h^{-1}} = 0.71\,h$$

At 6 h, the drug has been given for 8.5 half-lives and, thus, $C_P^6 \approx C_{SS}$ (see Section 2.1.2).

Equation (2.23): $C_{SS} = \frac{R}{V_D \cdot k} = \frac{R}{Cl_T}$ or $Cl_T = \frac{R}{C_{SS}} = \frac{380\,mg/h}{17.4\,mg/l} = 21.8\,l/h = 363\,ml/min$

$$Cl_T = V_D \cdot k \Rightarrow V_D = \frac{Cl_T}{k} = \frac{21.8\,l/h}{0.97\,h^{-1}} = 22.5\,l$$

7.14

The duration of the immediate-release tablets is only about 4.5 h, whereas that of the sustained-release tablets is over 12 h. The sustained-release tablets allow for administration every 12 h while the immediate-release tablets have to be administered every 5 h (i.e., they are difficult to administer). The immediate-release tablets result in much greater C_P fluctuation and greater risk of toxic side effects and lack of therapeutic effect. The sustained-release tablets result in much less C_P fluctuations and are much less likely to result in toxic side effects when taken every 12 h. Since these sustained-release tablets can be administered twice a day and are much less likely to cause toxic side effects, better patient compliance will generally be observed with sustained-release tablets compared with immediate-release tablets.

7.15

Cimetidine inhibits the hepatic metabolism of warfarin, thus increasing its anticoagulant effect. The dose should be reduced by about 50%, to $D_0 = 2.5$ mg and $\tau = 24$ h. Blood clotting time should be monitored in patients receiving warfarin.

7.16

Estimate the terminal half-life from the graph.

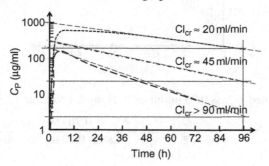

From Eq. (2.6):

$$\text{Cl}_{\text{Cr}} > 90 \text{ ml/min: } k = \frac{\ln\left(C_P^0/C_P\right)}{t} = \frac{\ln\left(200/2\right)}{96 \text{ h}} = 4.8 \cdot 10^{-2} \text{ h}^{-1}$$

$$\text{Cl}_{\text{Cr}} \approx 45 \text{ ml/min: } k = \frac{\ln\left(C_P^0/C_P\right)}{t} = \frac{\ln\left(300/20\right)}{96 \text{ h}} = 2.8 \cdot 10^{-2} \text{ h}^{-1}$$

$$\text{Cl}_{\text{Cr}} \approx 20 \text{ ml/min: } k = \frac{\ln\left(C_P^0/C_P\right)}{t} = \frac{\ln\left(900/200\right)}{96 \text{ h}} = 1.6 \cdot 10^{-2} \text{ h}^{-1}$$

Eq. (5.4) (same average plasma concentration):

$$\text{Cl}_{\text{Cr}} \approx 45 \text{ ml/min: } D_0' = D_0 \cdot \frac{k'}{k} = 666 \text{ mg} \cdot \frac{2.8 \cdot 10^{-2} \text{ h}^{-1}}{4.8 \cdot 10^{-2} \text{ h}^{-1}}$$

$$\approx 388 \text{ mg given every 8 h}$$

$$\text{Cl}_{\text{Cr}} \approx 20 \text{ ml/min: } D_0' = D_0 \cdot \frac{k'}{k} = 666 \text{ mg} \cdot \frac{1.6 \cdot 10^{-2} \text{ h}^{-1}}{4.8 \cdot 10^{-2} \text{ h}^{-1}}$$

$$\approx 222 \text{ mg given every 8 h}$$

7.17

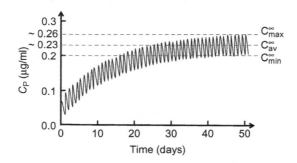

The estimated C_{av}^{∞} is 0.23 µg/ml or 0.23 mg/l. From Eq. (2.135), we get:

$$C_{\text{av}}^{\infty} = \frac{F \cdot D_0}{V_D \cdot k \cdot \tau} \Rightarrow k = \frac{F \cdot D_0}{V_D \cdot C_{\text{av}}^{\infty} \cdot \tau} \Rightarrow k = \frac{0.70 \cdot 50 \text{ mg}}{4{,}901 \cdot 0.23 \text{ mg/l} \cdot 1 \text{ day}} = 0.31 \text{ day}^{-1}$$

$$t_{\frac{1}{2}} = \frac{\ln 2}{0.31 \text{ day}^{-1}} = 2.2 \text{ days}$$

Since we do not have information about k_a, we will use the IV equation (Eq. (2.131)) to estimate the loading dose:

$$D_L = \frac{D_0}{1 - e^{-k \cdot \tau}} = \frac{50 \text{ mg}}{1 - e^{-0.31 \cdot 1}} \approx 190 \text{ mg}$$

Or we can estimate D_L from $C_{\text{max}}^{\infty} \approx 0.26$ mg/l:

$$D_L = \frac{C_{\text{max}}^{\infty} \cdot V_D}{F} \approx \frac{0.26 \cdot 490}{0.70} = 180 \text{ mg}$$

Appendix II

Symbols and Abbreviations

a first-order rate constant for the distribution phase

ADME absorption, distribution, metabolism, and excretion

ADME/Tox ADME and toxicology

API active pharmaceutical ingredient (i.e., the drug)

AUC area under the plasma concentration–time curve

b first-order rate constant for the elimination phase

β fraction of protein-bound drug

BCS Biopharmaceutics Classification System

BDDCS Biopharmaceutics Drug Disposition Classification System

C_a drug concentration in arterial plasma

C_{av}^{∞} average steady-state plasma drug concentration

C_{dt} hypothetical drug deep tissue concentration

C_{eff} minimum effective concentration (MEC)

Cl_B biliary clearance

Cl_{cr} creatinine clearance

Cl_D clearance in an artificial kidney machine (dialysis clearance)

Cl_H hepatic clearance

Cl_{inulin} inulin clearance

Cl_{NR} nonrenal clearance

Cl_R renal clearance

Cl_T total body clearance

C_{max} maximum plasma concentration (or peak plasma concentration)

C_P plasma concentration

C_P^0 plasma concentration at time 0

C_S drug solubility in water

C_{SS} steady-state plasma concentration

C_t hypothetical drug tissue concentration

C_v drug concentration in venous plasma

D diffusion coefficient

D:S dose–solubility ratio

D_0 amount of drug in body at time $(t) = 0$ (the drug dose)

D_B total amount of drug within the body

D_{dt} amount of drug in deep tissue compartment

D_e drug eliminated

D_{GI} drug dose in the GI tract

D_{IN} intranasal drug dose
D_{IV} intravenous drug dose
D_L loading dose
D_M maintenance dose
D_P amount of drug in central compartment
D-R drug–receptor complex
D_t amount of drug in tissue compartment
D_U amount of unmetabolized drug in urine
D_U^∞ amount of unmetabolized drug in urine at $t = \infty$
E enzyme
E pharmacologic effect (drug effect)
ED_{50} minimum effective dose for 50% of a population
ER liver extraction ratio
ES enzyme–substrate complex
F absolute (bio)availability
F_{bio} biologic availability
f_e fraction of drug excreted unchanged in urine
F_{pharm} pharmaceutical availability
F_{rel} relative (bio)availability
f_{ss} fraction of steady-state
f_u fraction of unbound drug
GFR glomerular filtration rate
GI gastrointestinal
h_D thickness of a UWL
h_M thickness of a membrane
IM intramuscular
IN intranasal
IV intravenous
η viscosity
J drug flux
k first-order elimination rate constant
k_0 zero-order rate constant for drug absorption
k_{12} first-order transfer rate constant from compartment 1 to compartment 2
k_{21} first-order transfer rate constant from compartment 2 to compartment 1
k_a first-order rate constant for drug absorption
k_b first-order rate constant for biliary excretion
k_e first-order rate constant for renal excretion
k_m first-order rate constant for drug metabolism
K_m Michaelis–Menten constant
$K_{M/D}$ partition coefficient between the membrane and the UWL (mucus)
k_{nr} first-order nonrenal rate constant
k_{rel} drug release rate constant from a formulation
LD_{50} lethal drug dose for 50% of an animal population
MEC minimum effective concentration
MTC minimum toxic concentration
M_w molecular weight
N Avogadro's number
NCE new chemical entity

OTC over-the-counter
P_D drug permeation coefficient through an UWL
per oral oral administration
per os oral administration
P_M drug permeation coefficient through a membrane
PO oral administration
$P_{o/w}$ octanol−water partition coefficient
PR rectal (per rectum)
P_T drug permeability through biomembranes such as the GI mucosa
Q blood flow
Q_{plasma} plasma flow through kidneys or liver
R zero-order drug infusion rate
R molar gas constant
R_D permeation resistance of an aqueous diffusion layer
RET rapidly equilibrating tissues
R_M permeation resistance of a membrane
SC subcutaneous
SET slowly equilibrating tissues
SL sublingual
t time
T absolute temperature
τ time interval between drug doses
$t_{1/2}$ half-life
$t_{1/2b}$ (or $t_{1/2\beta}$) drug half-life in the elimination phase (in two-compartment model)
TD$_{50}$ drug dose that produces toxicity in 50% of a population
TDM therapeutic drug monitoring
t_{eff} duration of drug action
TI therapeutic index
t_L lag time
t_m time midpoint of urine collection
t_{max} time at which C_{max} is observed
t_p time at which C_{max} is observed after multiple oral dosing
UWL unstirred water layer (sometimes referred to as an *aqueous diffusion layer*)
V_D apparent volume of distribution
$(V_D)_{area}$ apparent volume of distribution by area
$(V_D)_{exp}$ extrapolated volume of distribution
$(V_D)_{ss}$ apparent volume of distribution at steady-state
V_{dt} apparent volume of deep tissue compartment
V_{max} maximum velocity
V_P apparent volume of central compartment
V_t apparent volume of tissue compartment
∞ infinity

Index

Note: Page numbers followed by "*b*", "*f*", and "*t*" refer to boxes, figures, and tables, respectively.

Printed in the United States
By Bookmasters

Printed in the United States
By Bookmasters